Fitter Than Ever at 50 and Beyond

Susan Dawson-Cook, M.S.

Fitter Than Ever at 50 and Beyond
Copyright © 2021 Susan Dawson-Cook
ISBN: 9798529061015
Published by Corazon del Oro Communications, LLC
Cover Art by Anya Kelleye
Cover Photo by Laurie Slawson

ACKNOWLEDGEMENTS

I am forever grateful to Dr. Ellen Paige, Christopher Ferko, and Pat Dawson for their editorial and copy-editing assistance. A special thank you to Wally McKinzie, Barbara Stahura, Marilyn Krause, Mona Stanbrough, and Nancy Patchell Knoll for giving me permission to share their stories.

DISCLAIMER

This book offers ideas on how to improve fitness, lose weight and eat healthier. The content provided in this book is offered for informational purposes and should not be considered as medical advice, diagnosis or treatment. Always consult with your physician before starting an exercise program. Talk with your doctor before making dietary changes to ensure they are suitable for your current health status.

TABLE OF CONTENTS

INTRODUCTION

The *Fitter Than Ever* program yields outstanding results with work and commitment. I have no wand I can wave to melt off the weight and make your muscles strong (although I would wave one for you if I had one, believe me)! Instead, I offer a practical and healthy weight loss and maintenance program. I've formulated this plan through my own weight-loss journey, working with hundreds of personal training clients, and by studying research conducted by physicians and PhDs in the health and fitness field.

I published *Fitter Than Ever at 40 and Beyond* in 2017. The basic principles I outlined in that book are shared in this one. I have updated the information to include the latest apps and research and have added additional material. My life has evolved a great deal since the writing of my previous book. I have learned from personal experience and from working with many 50-something clients that during this phase of our lives, priorities and lifestyles shift. For this reason, I have added new chapters that are timely and relevant to many individuals in their fifties.

The *Fitter Than Ever* (whether at 40 or 50 or 100) program is not a diet—it is a change in lifestyle. The program will be effective if you maintain a high level of low to moderate activity and consume a reasonable amount of healthy food.

This program isn't about losing 50 pounds that you will promptly gain back weeks later. People who lose weight on fad diet plans only get slimmer because for a while, they eat fewer calories than are burned. That's the basic math of weight loss. You eat 500 to 750 calories less than you burn and you will lose at least one pound per week. It doesn't matter whether those calories come from chocolate or organic fruits and vegetables (although eating the wrong foods can make you experience unnecessary and uncomfortable cravings and hunger); the weight loss equation is basically about calories in and out.

The quality of your diet (whole, fresh foods versus sweets and junk food calories) will make a phenomenal difference in your ability to gain muscle and to control your cravings. That's why the *Fitter Than Ever* program is built on a foundation of healthy eating, rather than weird food combinations (and uncomfortable restrictions).

Why do people gain weight back once the fad diet ends? It's simple. After they can no longer tolerate subsisting on only chicken broth or fruit or eating pre-packaged meals, they revert to their "normal" eating habits again. The fad diet never helped them learn to eat in a sustainable way. "Normal" eating for most people involves excessively large portions and too much processed food.

America has become famous for its supersized portions to the point that most people don't know the difference between a "normal" and an "oversized" serving. Go to almost any restaurant today and they'll serve you as much as four times what you should be eating. By preparing food yourself, you will learn about how many calories are in different portions and begin to take control over your ability to lose or maintain your weight!

Following my healthy lifestyle plan, you will eat the same foods once you reach your ideal weight as you do after your initial food tracking stage. You will simply add more healthy food items to your diet to maintain your weight for life. If you've recently lost weight following another program, you can follow the *Fitter Than Ever* program from now on, so you can maintain your new weight indefinitely.

This program works. In *Fitter Than Ever at 40 and Beyond*, I shared my story and the stories of several clients who lost weight and improved their fitness and quality of life through my program.

Here's a short synopsis of my story. You've heard of the freshman 10? Well for me, it turned out to be the sophomore 25. When I stopped swimming competitively in college, I gained weight quickly and experienced constant hunger because I was accustomed to eating lots of food to accommodate the four hours of training I did almost daily. I also had some bad college student habits—weekend drinking binges, late night pizza ordering, and comfort M & Ms at hand while cramming for tests.

Initially, I found losing weight nearly impossible. I would pop diet pills, embark on fad diets and yo-yo between fasting and feasting. I woke up many nights after dreaming about food, overwhelmed by uncomfortable hunger.

Once I got back to basics—reading about nutrition, eating a better-balanced diet, trimming back alcohol intake, and finding exercise I found enjoyable (aerobic dance classes)—losing weight and maintaining it became easy. Over the course of two years, I lost 25 pounds without feeling deprived or experiencing gnawing hunger pains. From then on maintaining a healthy weight became pretty much effortless. I'd changed my lifestyle and maintaining my weight was about continuing with what I'd newly become accustomed to.

At age 58, I weigh what I did at age 16. As I just briefly mentioned, I haven't always been at my ideal weight or had a positive body image. I've experienced major struggles in both areas, which I'll share in more detail later. Many of us have these stories, these obstacles that impede our paths to a healthy lifestyle. Whether we choose to remain stuck or take steps to overcome these obstacles is a matter of choice. I can assure you that success is possible. You just have to believe in yourself and then put your head down and do the work that it takes to get there!

I recently retired from my work as a personal trainer. I now spend my days swimming in the Sea of Cortez (since I spend much of the year in San Carlos, Mexico), teaching yoga, volunteering with a sea turtle rescue group, and writing. Fitness plays a major role in my work and personal life. I carefully plan meals and rarely eat at restaurants. My husband is very athletic, so we often exercise together.

The positive benefits I reap from an active lifestyle motivate me to keep moving. Many people my age (and even as much as ten years younger) say they "used to" be an athlete or enjoy this or that activity. I find that tragic. No matter how busy you get, you deserve to take time out for activities that make you feel youthful and that preserve your health! As the years pass, it becomes more difficult to get in shape and or to perform the activities of daily living comfortably when you live sedentary. Joints stiffen, muscle mass and aerobic fitness decline—and regaining what is lost becomes more difficult with every passing year.

It is possible to be active the rest of your life even if your schedule is crazy. I'll share my story later of how I stayed fit when my work as a sales manager required me to travel fifty percent of the time.

And you can keep moving even if you are experiencing physical limitations. You might have to modify the intensity or the way you exercise as years pass. Most of us do. I had to give up running triathlons six years ago after suffering an injury to my sacroiliac that recurred whenever I started running too often again. An illness or surgical procedure may even mean taking a hiatus from exercise. Bed rest was prescribed to me for two (very long) months when I was pregnant with my son.

I now only run on the track, flat beach, or trails (or Woodway treadmills) because running on pavement or hard treadmill surfaces irritates my knees and sacroiliac joint. Once a week I take a day of complete rest. If my shoulder hurts during a swim, I change strokes or start kicking, but never push through it and make it worse. Since I tore my right rotator cuff in 2008 (and successfully rehabilitated it with the help of a physical therapist), I have had to be especially careful not to do crazy things with my shoulders. Activities I have to be especially cautious about are excessive swimming, kayaking, volleyball, and loaded hands-above-shoulders movements (such as an overhead press with weights or putting a heavy suitcase in an overhead bin on a plane). By getting to know your body (and listening to its cues), you can avoid unnecessary injuries and lost exercise time.

There are many other ways I modify activity on almost a daily basis, which mostly involve listening to body cues and using information I know about my own body to do what's practical. Learning to understand what works and doesn't work for your body instead of forcing it into submission will enable you to enjoy your favorite activities indefinitely. The information I will share with you from my thirty-plus years working on the ground as a fitness professional will support your efforts.

Rumor has it if you're over fifty and slender you live on carrot sticks, exercise four hours a day or have an eating disorder. People often say I look great before they ask if I exercise four hours a day (I don't) or if I eat anything except broccoli.

The truth is I don't take weight loss pills, diuretics, dine on only raw vegetables, or follow ridiculous diet plans (been there, done that and I'm definitely not going to do it again). I have in recent years by choice eliminated grains, alcohol and sugar from my diet. I made this choice for health reasons (better digestion and neurological functioning) and not to change my weight—which was already where I wanted it before I made this change.

You, too, can exercise and eat your way into fitting into clothes you haven't worn for years that are collecting dust in the back of your closet. Within days of following the *Fitter Than Ever* program, you'll have more energy, lose pounds and inches, and feel increasingly motivated to continue.

You don't have to starve yourself to be slender. You watch people sweating on the treadmill and in the weight room for 8 hours a day on "The Biggest Loser" and imagine only all-day workouts and a rice cake diet will shrink you enough for you to fit into a size 6 skirt. Not true. In reality, these "boot camp" diet plans slow your metabolism and predispose you to eventually regaining all that weight. I know, because I tried dozens of boot camp diet plans during my college days and ended up heavier every time. This book offers you strategies for losing weight and keeping it off for life!

You will eat "like a normal person," although we may have to reestablish a baseline for "normal." "Normal" portions in America tend to mean most of the day's calories get consumed in one meal. This has to change if you want to lose weight. I'll elaborate on this later, but in a nutshell, it means you can eat a variety of foods, but that you must limit the amount, that you can have dessert, but not too often, that you can have an alcoholic beverage, but only one and not every night.

What you will avoid like the plague is the sedentary lifestyle of the "normal person." Because that is a behavior pattern I can only describe as "button-bursting." Some of you will find—as I did—that certain foods irritate your digestive system or trigger cravings or uncomfortable hunger. You may want to eliminate those. Figuring this out will involve some trial and error.

Unlike the contestants on weight loss reality shows, you will have time for your family and your job. My goal is to help you make moderate exercise and healthy eating a permanent part of your lifestyle. You will "live right" day after day until healthy living becomes as much of a daily habit as putting on deodorant and brushing your teeth.

Regular exercise and eating a healthy diet mean much more than a slimmer body. They have been proven to reduce your risk for heart disease, diabetes, cancer and a host of other longevity stealing illnesses.[1] A 1993 study by McGinnis and Foege showed that eighty percent of premature deaths in the U.S. are connected to dietary patterns, physical activity level (or lack of it) and tobacco use.[2] It is completely within your grasp to have more energy, less pain, and better health just by changing your diet and moving more. Isn't it worth it?

I'm not saying I've never slipped away from proper exercise and eating and that's why I'm thin. Exactly the opposite. I was once at rock bottom with my eating habits and self-esteem. If you're there now, you don't have to stay there. I've left behind all those negative thoughts and formed a new attitude about weight and body image. Now I have a harmonious relationship with my body. I'm strong and fit and flexible and move with ease. I know that you can experience all of these benefits, too, if you give yourself the chance. Embark with me on a new journey.

Once I persuade you to ditch the fad-dieting rollercoaster and focus on health, you can begin to eat foods that reduce your disease risk. You will work more activity into your daily schedule, start reading (and analyzing) food labels, and shun foods loaded with preservatives and sugar that lead to weight gain and poor health. It's really quite simple.

Within days, you'll have more energy and feel more optimistic. As these positive benefits of your new lifestyle continue to build, you will experience better health, a leaner profile, and more ease and enjoyment of favorite activities and sports. Thank you for taking this journey with me to better health and wellness. Helping people live well brings me a great deal of joy and fulfillment.

REFERENCES

1 - Hu, F.B., J.E. Manson, M.J. Stampfer, G. Colditz, S. Liu, C.G. Solomon, and W. C. Willett. 2001. "Diet, lifestyle, and the risk of type 2 diabetes mellitus in women." *N Engl J Med* 345(11); 790-797.

2 - McGinnis, Michael, and William Foege. 1993. "Actual Causes of Death in the United States." *JAMA*. 270 (18): 2207-2212.

CHAPTER ONE

The Fitter Than Ever Program

There are seven components of the *Fitter than Ever* program designed to help you succeed. You will need to purchase a journal to record information on each of these seven areas so you can track your progress and find ways to overcome roadblocks. This journal will be where you record numbers and data and also strategize and free write about your experiences and what's working and what's not working. The seven components of this are:

1) **Your Goals.** You will establish realistic, specific, and measurable goals.

2) **Your Exercise Plan** (which includes A. Aerobic/cardiovascular conditioning and B. Strength training). If lack of flexibility is inhibiting your ability to do activities you enjoy, you may want to add stretching or yoga to your program. If you are coping with stress and anxiety,

yoga and/or meditation are good options. Managing stress often makes it easier to eat healthy.

3) **Your Healthy Eating Plan,** which is not a "diet" and does not limit the consumption of any foods or beverages other than the ones most harmful to your health. You will keep a food journal, evaluate the problem areas and begin to (when appropriate) reduce caloric intake.

4) **Your Tracking Plan**. You will record some baseline information so you can track your progress.

5) **Your Lifestyle Plan.** This will involve becoming aware of lifestyle habits (too little sleep, late afternoon munchies, skipping meals, mindless or stress eating, etc.) that are inhibiting progress. You will make permanent modifications to these behaviors for the better. In your journal, you will write down strategies you plan to employ to increase your chance of success.

6) **Your Motivation Plan.** You will exercise with a friend, spouse (or adopt a dog you will enjoy walking with), join group exercise classes, or embark on activities such as walkathons, triathlons, cycling rides, depending on what motivates you most. Maybe you want to post a photo of someone with your goal physique on your refrigerator!

7) **Your Follow Susan's Slim For Life Secrets Plan.** These "secrets" work amazingly well for me and countless others who lost weight and kept it off. By adding these to your bag

of tricks, you will be able to achieve your goal of permanent weight loss, which comes from living a healthy lifestyle.

1) **Your Goals**

Most people who make New Year's resolutions pertaining to weight loss and exercise never outline a plan on how they will accomplish that objective. This dooms them to failure. If you want to adopt a new healthy lifestyle, you have to make a commitment to it and you have to have a plan to get from point A (dissatisfied with health, physical conditioning, and weight) to point B (your goal weight, improved energy level, aerobic fitness, strength, etc.).

Write down a list of SMART goals in your journal. These must be Specific, Measurable, Attainable (realistic), Relevant (rewarding) and Trackable. I want to lose weight is not a SMART goal. I want to lose 25 pounds by May 25th for my daughter's graduation is an example of a smart goal. If you want to lower cholesterol, establish a number you would like to achieve. Are there any medications you would like to stop taking? (Please consult with your physician before stopping any medications).

I suggest recording both short-term and long-term goals to stay motivated. One short-term goal could be to increase weekly aerobic exercise from 10 minutes a day to 30 minutes a day by the end of the month. Make sure goals are realistic.

It isn't sustainable to lose more than two pounds a week, so keep this in mind when you record weight loss goals.

2) **Your Exercise Plan**

The information provided here is a guideline. Please consult with your physician to make sure it is safe for you to embark on an exercise program.

Daily activity will play a major role in helping you lose weight. It will also deliver many side benefits including increased energy, better mood, and improved sleep. Exercise is also a great stress buster. Make sure to block out time in your weekly schedule for both cardiovascular and strength training workouts as outlined below.

It's going to be tempting to skip workouts from time to time. In order to improve adherence, please always schedule workout times for the upcoming week on Sunday afternoon. Maybe you plan to take an exercise class Monday, Wednesday and Friday at 6 AM (or 8 AM if you're retired) and walk for an hour with a friend on Tuesday and Thursday evenings.

Schedule exercise sessions in your smart phone or day planner the same way you would enter a doctor's appointment! Select every class you will attend and/or block out the hours you will do your cardiovascular and strength training. Commit to only missing in the event of an actual emergency or illness. Recognize that if you embark on this "schedule," in a few months it will become a habit and less of a chore to maintain. You'll likely begin to look forward to your workouts.

Scheduling workouts ahead of time has been a lifesaver for me. I'm always thinking about which days I will swim, run, practice yoga or hike. If you build in time in your schedule for exercise, you will follow through and succeed at making activity part of your daily life.

It is crucial to listen to your body. Avoid jumping into too much activity too soon when your body is unprepared for it. Your body will slowly adapt as you increase activity level and intensity. Consider cross training with different forms of aerobic exercise to reduce excessive repetitive stress.

Most injuries happen when people take classes or dive into exercise too advanced for their current fitness levels or don't listen to body cues that, if tuned in to, could have prevented the injury. My approach is to train so I can continue being active well into my 80s. For example, if I wake up and notice one of my knees isn't moving freely without discomfort, I will choose to do a light- or non-impact activity (such as swimming or easy walking) over running or aerobics, which would be likely to aggravate the already vulnerable joint.

Exercise has become as much of a habit for me as brushing my teeth. I feel out-of-kilter all day when I miss a workout due to a plane trip or family emergency. If you've been sedentary for many years, it's going to take several months to break the temptation to return to the couch. You may hear all kinds of chatter in your head in the form of excuses. You don't listen to every temptation to buy something when you're at the mall, do you? Shut down these sabotaging thoughts. Push through and keep forging ahead toward your goals. It will be well worth it!

Once workouts become part of your routine, the time "lost" won't feel like a sacrifice anymore. Instead, it will feel like me-time, like an opportunity to renew your energy, refresh your mind and escape all of your responsibilities for a little while. Often my workout time is the most peaceful time in my day. Nothing thrills me more than my swims in the Sea of Cortez, when often a pod of bottlenose dolphins glide over to visit, circling around me, blowing bubbles and trying to communicate with squeaks and whistles. The experience of being outdoors and seeing the dolphins also makes me feel very connected to nature and the other beings that inhabit this planet with us — a very peaceful feeling.

A. Cardiovascular Training. Each week, accumulate a minimum of 250 minutes of cardiovascular/aerobic exercise. If you haven't done any aerobic exercise recently, start with a gentle 100 minutes per week and build up to 250 over the course of the next two months. Aerobic exercise includes anything *continuous* in nature (swimming, running, walking, hiking, cycling, rowing machine, treadmill, elliptical machine, etc.). Stop and start sports such as tennis, golf, racquetball and pickleball are great, but they are not continuous, fat-burning exercise and should not be counted toward your 250 minutes.

You can attend exercise classes such as spin, low-impact aerobics, dance classes (such as Zumba), water aerobics, or step, **counting only the continuous movement portions of the class toward your 250-minute weekly total**. The only exception to this would be a class with "interval training" where your heart rate stays elevated, strength segments use large muscle groups (thighs, chest and back), and transitions to different activities are rapid. You can count a full class like this toward your total minutes.

If you haven't found a modality of exercise you enjoy, experiment over the next 30 days. Try different sports and activities until you find something you like and that works for your body. Many people in their 50s find running uncomfortable. Don't force yourself to do something that isn't working for you or that is so unpleasant that it incites a negative attitude about your exercise program. Finding activity that you truly enjoy will enable you to look forward to being active and greatly increase your adherence.

To accumulate your 250 weekly minutes, you could engage in 50 minutes of walking, 5 days per week for example. You can do this in bouts of as short as 10 minutes if necessary, but fat burning doesn't really get started until 20 minutes or more of continuous movement (in the beginning your body relies on glycogen stored in the muscles).

Always increase intensity gradually, so your muscles and joints have a chance to properly warm-up. This will reduce the potential for a muscle strain or other uncomfortable symptoms. The warm-up period should be a minimum of 5 minutes and last up to 10 minutes if you haven't been exercising regularly or are over 50.

Always complete your workout with a cool down, gradually reducing the intensity so your blood can redistribute from working muscles to the rest of your body. This cool down period can make a big difference in how you feel post-workout. If you give your body time to recirculate blood and your heart rate to slowly decrease instead of jolting to a stop, you shouldn't feel lightheaded after activity. Gentle stretching for 5 to 10 minutes can restore length to tissues and can help you relax. I offer many stretch and yoga videos on my Vimeo page if you need some ideas (https://vimeo.com/ondemand/yogawithsusan). My Gentle Yoga classes are ideal for stretching and relaxation.

If you experience joint or muscle pain associated with arthritis, fibromyalgia or another condition, consider warm water exercise. Water aerobics, swimming or walking in water over 85 degrees relaxes the muscles and joints. Many individuals with osteoarthritis who experience nearly constant pain on land experience comfortable and free movement in the water. The combination of the heat, water, and motion is what helps so much. Waist-deep in water, a person carries only 50 percent of his/her body weight around. The reduction becomes even greater when in chest deep water and a person becomes virtually weightless suspended on a noodle or while swimming.

Initially, water exercise participants may only feel this amazing difference while in the aquatic environment but many that persist with this exercise modality notice the reduced joint and muscular pain and discomfort carries over to the rest of their day on dry land. [11,12]

It is beneficial to use a heart rate monitor during cardiovascular training workouts. Please note that your heart rate levels will be different when you exercise in the water. This can vary depending on water temperature and degree of submersion. It will be reasonably accurate to reduce your "land" target heart rates that you calculate by about 13 percent to adjust for this difference. You can do this by taking—for example—your 60 percent of maximum number and multiplying it by .87. If your 60 percent number were 100 beats per minute, for example, your new value for water training would be 87. [16]

Unless your physician offers different guidelines, aim to maintain an intensity between 60 and 80 percent of your maximum heart rate. A conservative estimated maximum heart rate can be most simply calculated by subtracting your age from 220. To obtain the 60 and 80 percent (of maximum heart rate) numbers that will comprise your training range, multiply that sum by .6 to get the 60 percent number and by .8 to get the 80 percent number.

As an example, I will show how to calculate these numbers for me (I'm 58 years old). My maximum heart rate would be 220 - 58 or 162. I avoid training close to my maximum heart rate because it could be dangerous. To calculate target ranges, I take 162 x .6 to get my 60 percent maximum heart rate number (97) and 162 x .8 to get my 80 percent maximum heart rate number (130). If you are new to exercise, train between 50 and 70 percent of maximum your first month and then gradually increase intensity as you feel more comfortable.

Please consult with your physician for guidelines if you have a heart condition. Some cardiac medications affect your resting (and training) heart rates, so it is best to use perceived exertion (described in more detail on the next page) as a guideline.

The 220 minus age estimate yields very low target heart rates for older adults. These limiting estimates will hinder very fit adults and athletes, who have the potential to train at significantly higher heart rates than unfit individuals of the same age.

If you've engaged in athletic training or regular cardiovascular training most of your life, have no cardiac risks, and are not taking high blood pressure medications, you should be able to safely go up to 80 to 85 percent of your maximum heart rate during training or a workout based on a less conservative estimate computed by subtracting 1/2 your age from 210.

More advanced exercisers—including athletes—can train at even higher intensities and heart rates. Intensity should be reduced (and in most instances, the workout ended) in all populations if dizziness, nausea, or irregular heart rhythms are experienced. The 5 Zones, and the individuals who can safely exercise within each of them, are explained in detail in Appendix I.

Most treadmills, ellipticals, and bicycles at fitness centers allow you to monitor heart rate by gripping handles with metal sensors for a period of time until a digital reading of your heart rate appears on the console.

While hiking, walking, cycling, and taking group exercise classes, wearing a heart rate monitor will make it possible for you to track exercise intensity. Heart rate monitors can be purchased online or at sporting goods stores. Although fancy models will reveal current altitude, predict the weather and allow you to download data to your computers and tablets, most people will do just fine with a basic model, which can be purchased for $100 or less.

Be sure to make sure the device matches your goals. For example, a Fitbit which measures daily steps and heart rate won't be very useful to a triathlete who will want downloadable data on distance and pace for different modalities of exercise.

Some possible options for heart rate monitors/watches are the Polar H10, Willful Smartwatch, Wahoo Fitness TICKR FIT, Fitbit Versa 2 Smartwatch, and Garmin HRM-Tri (works in water). The Garmin Swim Watch is good for tracking swimming distance but does not offer heartrate information. The Garmin Forerunner 935/945 works for all sports and does track heart rate.

If you take beta-blockers, calcium channel blockers and other (usually for cardiovascular disease) medications that lower heart rate, it is important that you exercise according to how you feel (perceived exertion), rather than going by a heart rate calculation (which might subject you to dangerously high heart rates).

This method of estimating exercise intensity, which has a scale that runs from 0 to 10, is known as the Rated Perceived Exertion Scale (RPE). A zero would be sitting in a chair immobile. A 2 to 3 on the RPE scale would be light activity that you can easily sustain for an hour or more, which would allow you to freely converse. A 4 out of 10 on the RPE scale (Somewhat Hard), would leave you breathing heavily, but still able to talk (see Appendix I for the RPE table).

Another very simple method you can utilize during cardiorespiratory training is known as the "Talk Test." If you are unable to speak at all while you exercise, you are working too hard. If you can chatter on incessantly, you need to step it up!

If you're in good cardiovascular health, aim to do a minimum of 60 of your 250 weekly minutes as "interval training" where you periodically increase and decrease intensity. The benefit of interval training is that you will burn more overall calories than doing steady-state activity and will get an increased caloric burn (above your resting metabolic rate or RMR) for hours after the workout compared to other forms of training.

For example, if you want to do a thirty-minute interval workout on the treadmill, I recommend that you warm up for 5 minutes, then do bouts of 4 minutes hard followed by 2 minutes at a slow pace for 4 cycles (total of 24 minutes) and then cool down for the last few minutes. You can do the hard intervals by either increasing treadmill speed or incline. On a bicycle, you can increase intensity by increasing rotations per minute (how fast you pedal) or resistance level. Some sample interval workouts can be found in Appendix II.

If possible, engage in at least one long steady session per week (a walk, hike, or swim of 60 or more minutes). Long duration, low intensity exercise burns more body fat than many other workouts. To determine how many calories are burned doing different activities, you can refer to https://www.healthstatus.com/calculate/cbc

Keep in mind that as your aerobic conditioning improves, you will need to gradually increase intensity to continue progressing. What once elevated your heart rate to 70 percent of MHR won't continue to do so as your heart and circulatory system becomes more efficient. Your body is a master at adapting to meet the demands you place on it.

Many people who walk daily get to the point where they no longer increase heart rate or break a sweat. This kind of halfhearted exercise will not improve cardiovascular fitness or Body Mass Index (BMI).

Losing weight requires that you keep upping the ante as your level of fitness improves. If you no longer sweat and can talk non-stop during your walk, it's time to step it up! Increase your tempo and swing your arms until you get your heart rate within that 60 to 80 percent of MHR level (using Rate of Perceived Exertion (RPE) instead when applicable).

Clients and friends experiencing a weight loss plateau often report that they "break through" the barrier by changing up their routine and giving their body a workout surprise.

Any change in your exercise program causes adaptive changes. Your body is constantly restructuring bone and muscle to accommodate stresses placed on it. For example, if you always walk on the treadmill for your cardio minutes, try working out on the elliptical for a week or two or attending a group exercise class once a week. Your body has to work harder to adapt to these changes.

Cross training, or embarking on different activities throughout each week, is even the best option because it minimizes the potential for repetitive stress injuries that can come from doing the same movement patterns day after day.

As your activity level increases, you will need to drink more water to stay properly hydrated. When exercising in very hot weather or extreme humidity (especially if running or hiking long distances), salt pills or electrolyte drinks may be beneficial or even necessary.

If possible, weigh yourself before and after exercise and drink enough water to raise your weight back to what it was pre-exercise. This will ensure you aren't dehydrated. If you feel hungry after your workout, drink water first. Sometimes thirst can be misinterpreted as hunger.

B. Strength Training. Each week, you will strength train a minimum of 2 days per week. Please rest at least 48 hours between sessions and warm up for at least five minutes before starting the session. For a basic program, you will do 2 sets of 10 to 12 repetitions for major muscle groups using one or more of the following: machines, free weights, stretch cords, weighted bars, weighted balls, and body weight. **If you are unsure how to strength train correctly, please consult with a certified personal trainer, choose a strength-oriented exercise class to attend (2 days per week) or do machine workouts after getting instructions from a gym**

attendant. Performing exercises too fast or incorrectly can lead to injury.

Inhale and exhale during each repetition. Exhale during the exertion phase of the repetition. Avoid locking your elbows or knees when in extension to reduce stress on the joints. Do the exercises slowly to reduce the potential for injury. Please embark on strength workouts conservatively (with light weights at first), especially if you're not accustomed to doing them. Muscle soreness may occur 24 to 48 hours after your training session, but if you experience soreness that interferes with sleep or daily living tasks, you are working too hard.

If you are new to strength training, it is safest to start with machines. Machines work most of your major muscle groups. The ones I mention below are available at most gyms and fitness centers. Machines usually have images posted on them, which show working muscles and sometimes include written instructions on how to perform the exercise safely. Many gyms offer a free introductory session with a basic explanation on how to adjust the machines to fit your height and limb length.

Start with a weight that challenges you and enables you to finish the set with good form. Do the exercises in a slow, controlled manner. Record the date, the name of the piece of equipment, the weight selected and any seat or apparatus settings on your exercise card. Continue to track your training and once the set starts to feel easy (you are able to easily do two or more reps beyond your normal set), you can increase the weight. Increase by no more than ten percent at a time.

1) Leg Press Machine – works quadriceps (front of thighs), hamstrings (back of thighs) and gluteus maximus (buttocks). Place feet hip width apart on platform. Keep knees and toes tracking forward. Avoid locking knees and do not allow plates to touch (or crash together) during the set.

2) Leg Curl Machine - works hamstrings. Adjust so knees line up with and move with the joint of the machine (sometimes there is a red dot in the center of the joint that makes it easier to check). Pull heels down until they are under the knees before slowly allowing heels to raise back up.

There is also a prone version of this machine available. Choose this one only if the seated machine isn't available. It is important not to arch your back or let your hips rise off of the pad when doing prone leg curls. This will tend to happen if you set the weight too high. Keep in mind since you are working against gravity in the prone position, you will need to select a lighter weight than you use for the seated version of this exercise.

3) Lat Pulldown Machine – works Latissimus Dorsi muscles in the back. Pull down leading with elbows until hands are at the level of your ears. Make sure your bottom stays down on the seat and do not use your lower back (jerking back or forward to enable yourself to lift more with momentum).

4) Seated Row – works middle back – Trapezius muscles. Sit up in tall posture, chest firm against the front pad, and lead with the elbows as you pull back. Retract the shoulder blades, imagining that you are allowing them to glide down the back. Keep shoulders down and away from the ears. Make sure there is resistance throughout the range of motion (you will need to adjust your distance from the handles to further away if you don't have a full range of motion without the plates touching).

5) Chest Press – works pectorals, biceps and triceps. Avoid locking your elbows and avoid allowing the elbows to drop behind shoulders, which can strain or tear internal rotators.

6) Arm curl (there is one for biceps, another for triceps); your elbow should move with the joint of the machine.

7-8) Abduction/Adduction machine – works inner and outer thighs (there are usually 2 different machines, although sometimes there is a machine where you flip the pads around to work the different set of muscles). Pads are placed on the outside of thigh to work the outer thighs and on the inside of thighs to work inner thighs. Avoid arching your back when you do abduction (outer thigh) work. Be careful about using too much weight or widening your legs open too far to start on the adduction (inner thigh) exercise. These muscles are very susceptible to injury.

Optional: Abdominal exercises. Strengthening the abdominal muscles builds a strong core, which means you will have better balance, posture and stability during different activities. Be sure to train the internal and external obliques (side abs) and the transverse abdominals (deeper abs) in addition to the rectus abdominus (central abs).

Please keep in mind when you do ab work that you can't shrink your belly or any other part of your body by working it to death. I don't know how this spot-reducing rumor got started, but after 35 years in the fitness industry, people still ask me about it and are surprised to learn it just isn't so! If you have a flabby belly, you will have to burn off the fat by doing cardiovascular training and eating less. Even if you do 500 crunches a day, if the fat isn't burned off, your stomach won't look any flatter and no one will ever see your toned muscles!

I do not recommend abdominal machines as they load these endurance muscles too heavily and may lead to injury. I also do not recommend full sit-ups because they work the hip flexors more than the abdominals and can irritate or possibly injure the spine.

It is safest to do simple abdominal exercises on a mat or ball. Do 12 to 20 repetitions for each abdominal exercise you do using only body weight (no machine weight). Options – bicycles, reverse curls, quarter crunches, diagonal crunches, etc. You can also do planks, holding the position for several breaths. Make sure to keep the neck lengthened. You can do front or side planks down on your forearms if you have wrist issues.

A good exercise for spinal health is the bird dog. Begin on your hands and knees and extend your right arm straight out (thumb up), your left leg straight back (heel no higher than the hip) and then lower them and then do the same thing with the left arm/right leg and repeat that 12 times. Pull the belly up slightly during the activity so your lower back doesn't sag and keep your head in alignment with the rest of your spine.

If you want to strength train at home, you can order almost any fitness equipment you need including stability balls, dumbbells (hand weights), resistance bands, weighted bars, medicine balls, kettle balls, BOSU balls, gliding disks, yoga mats, etc. from power-systems.com.

*Osteoporosis Note: If you have osteoporosis, you should avoid exercising (or household activities) that involve twisting and unsupported forward flexion (leaning forward unanchored to something), both of which have been linked to spinal fractures.

* **Falling Hazard Note:** While exercising at home, be careful about leaving equipment in the middle of the floor because it can be a tripping hazard.

Summary of Exercise Points

- Do 250 minutes of Aerobic Exercise per week
- Do 2 Strength Training Workouts per week, working major muscle groups
- Pre-Plan Workout times
- Work at Appropriate Level by Tracking Heart Rate
- Make Exercise a Healthy Habit

3) Your Healthy Eating Plan

I can almost hear you saying, "oh no," but please don't panic. I don't expect you to starve yourself, live off of raw vegetables or turn up the music volume to drown out hungry tummy growls. This program is all about being mindful of food consumption, making healthier choices, and employing eating strategies that help you lose weight and keep it off. You'll also feel empowered because you will be in control of what you're eating instead of allowing television ads, food company displays in grocery stores, and cravings to drive your choices.

Food fuels your body. When you eat a nutrient-poor diet, you may feel achy, fatigued and lethargic, have trouble concentrating, feel stressed out more often, and be more susceptible to illness. Start eating more nutritious food and you'll be surprised at how much healthier, happier, and even smarter you feel.

Your first step is to keep a food journal for two weeks in your *Fitter Than Ever* journal, eating as normally as possible and listing every single item eaten and every beverage consumed.

For the sake of simplicity, the energy value of food and drinks or kilocalories will be referred to as calories in this book since what you see on food labels—actually kilocalories—appear as "calories."

Record portions and total calories for the meal or snack as accurately as possible. You might want to buy a digital scale to weigh your food, or you can use measuring cups. You can estimate calories by looking up foods at www.dietbites.com/Calories-Simple-Foods/ or using one of the many calorie-counting apps available today on your smart phone or tablet. Fitbit, HealthyOut, NutritionIx, and

MyFitnessPal are some phone apps you can use to track calories and eating.

Please be very specific about portions. Many clients have put down wine or rice instead of 4-ounce glass of wine or 1/2 cup of rice. The difference in calories between 1/2 cup and 1 cup of a food is significant as is one glass of wine compared to the whole bottle! I don't expect you to go to your neighborhood parties with a measuring cup in hand so here's a trick you can use. Begin by measuring liquids and pouring it in a wine or drinking glass to learn to fairly accurately estimate drink amounts.

To estimate quantity of dry foods, fill a measuring cup up to 1/2 cup with dry cereal or lentils and then pour that on a plate. Try this again with 1 cup and then 1 1/2 and then 2. Get an idea of how much food you are eating by looking at these quantities so you will be able to reasonably accurately assess portion size on the go.

At the end of the 2 weeks, you will analyze your food chart for "trouble spots" and begin to follow a restricted calorie plan based on your computed RMR (resting metabolic rate) and TDEE (total daily energy requirement) as outlined in the next section. You will want to track the number of calories you are consuming and also make sure that you are eating a healthy balance of foods. In general, you will want to eat fresh foods—especially vegetables and fruits. Everyone's body thrives on a slightly different combination of macronutrients so being in tune with this will help you find a nutritional formula that you feel comfortable with. It will be helpful for you to identify the following dietary hazards: 1) meal skipping, 2) excessive alcohol consumption, 3) midnight snacking, 4) consumption of empty calories (sodas, chips, sugary snacks), 5) mindless eating (in front of the TV, in the car, etc.), 6) stress/emotional eating, 7) eating excessively at parties or restaurants and 8) eating when you're not hungry.

All of these may lead to you eating more calories per day than you're burning. Continue with that pattern and your weight will continue to climb with every passing year! That's why you want to get a handle on these issues now. Then you can halt weight gain and start to move the scale in a downward direction instead!

In your Goals section, go back and outline some strategies you will implement to avoid these pitfalls. At regular intervals, you will go back to this page and make notes about how your strategies are working and modify them if necessary.

Determine RMR and Goal Caloric intake for Weight Loss

All of us have a basal metabolic rate (BMR), or energy amount (usually measured in number of calories) that we need to survive in a state of rest every 24 hours. When most of us think of metabolism, we think of the breakdown of food particles and its transformation into energy, but metabolism encompasses a range of biochemical processes within our bodies. Metabolism consists both of anabolism and catabolism; the buildup and breakdown of substances, respectively.

Metabolic energy is expended for breathing, blood circulation, body temperature regulation, cell growth, brain and nerve function, and muscle contractions.[2,9] If you want the most accurate number, you can have your BMR or RMR measured. Determining RMR or Resting Metabolic Rate is easier than BMR (BMR is usually measured in a dark room immediately after wakening; RMR does not require the patient to sleep overnight in a facility). To get this test done, you will need to consult with a nutrition specialist or exercise physiologist that has the required equipment.

You can obtain an *estimate* of BMR/RMR by entering your height, weight, age and sex on this website (http://www.etoolsage.com/Calculator/BMR_Calculator.asp?toolsort=1500). Most people have an RMR between 800 and 1500 Kilocalories. According to this site (Harris-Benedict formula), my RMR is 1174 calories.

Despite how unfair it seems some people can eat more than others without gaining weight. If you weigh more, which means you might be male, taller or be carrying abundant pounds of muscle, fat or both, you will burn more calories than a smaller person. This means that a man can eat more than a woman without gaining weight and that a tall or larger-framed woman can eat more than a more petite woman without gaining weight.

RMR and BMR tend to decrease with age (at a rate of about 1 to 2 percent per decade after age 20) as lean muscle tissue declines. Metabolic rates can be affected for better or worse by muscle mass, body temperature, health, glandular function, and diet (skipping meals and overly restricting calories can also cause BMR to decrease). [4]

Strength training is key to maintaining calorie-burning muscle mass. If you halt the loss of muscle mass, you will burn more calories and be able to eat more without weight gain than someone of the same sex of similar weight who has less muscle mass.

Use your measured or estimated Resting Metabolic Rate (RMR) and an activity level multiplier (known as the Harris-Benedict multipliers) as a basis to estimate your daily calorie requirement. Keep in mind that these multipliers should be selected based on the amount of time you spend exercising and how active you are the rest of the day.

To keep things simple, you will use the following formulas to estimate your total daily energy requirement (TDEE) or the number of calories you require to maintain your weight **(RMR x exercise multiplier) = Required calories for weight maintenance.** Your goal should be to do moderate or more intense exercise (if appropriate) most days of the week. **To lose a pound per week, you will want to eat your computed TDEE calories - 500. You may use TDEE - 750 if you want to lose weight faster and are able to do this without uncomfortable hunger pangs.**

Any day you skip exercise and are generally sedentary (watching TV, sitting in front of the computer, driving); you will multiply your RMR x 1.2 to compute your caloric requirement for that day. For example, let's go back to my RMR of 1174 calories. I multiply that number by 1.2, giving me a total of 1408 calories, the number of calories I need to eat to maintain my weight on a day I do no activity. **To stay on the one pound per week weight loss goal, I would eat 909 calories on a light activity day.** That isn't very much food! Now you can see why exercise is so important.

Any day you are lightly active (do some house or yard work or walk your dog with multiple stops for example), your multiplier will be 1.375. Using my RMR, my caloric requirement on a light activity day becomes 1614.25.

Any day you exercise at least 30 minutes at a moderate intensity and are generally active throughout the day, your multiplier will be 1.55.

Any day you exercise more than an hour at a high intensity (over 70 percent of MHR), your multiplier will be 1.725. Using my RMR, my break-even caloric requirement now becomes a much more comfortable 2025 calories!

Any day you participate in high intensity exercise or athletic training (for an hour or more) and work at a very physical job, your multiplier will be 1.9.

Make sure you use multipliers that apply for what you're actually doing, not what you aim to do in the future. Avoid choosing a high multiplier on a day you exercised and then crashed the rest of the day on the sofa. It is always better to go conservative on the TDEE estimates in the beginning until you start losing weight and better understand your body's energy requirements.

You can see from these calculations that if I were inactive all the time, I would have to eat a very restrictive diet to maintain my weight. That's why many people who don't overeat end up overweight.

By upping the ante on my activity level, which I do almost daily, caloric intake numbers that sans activity were very low and could make me feel frustrated or discouraged increased significantly, so maintaining my weight became easy rather than a struggle. It is to your advantage to exercise more because it allows you to eat more. For years, I have simply eaten healthy food whenever I'm hungry and have had no struggle with weight. No struggle at all. I wrote this book because I want that same thing to happen for you!

Now record what you're eating for two more weeks. For best results, I recommend tracking everything you eat until you have reached your desired weight and maintained it for at least six months. It's very easy to track food nowadays in Apps, especially once you get all of your common foods entered into the program. Once healthy eating becomes a habit, you can pursue your new way of eating without tracking as long as your weight stays stable.

During this two-week period and beyond, please adhere to the following guidelines:

1) *No meal skipping.* If you've never eaten breakfast, please start now. It's fine to have a small portion, such as a piece of fruit or 1/2 cup of yogurt but eat some kind of breakfast so you don't end up overeating later. Every day you will eat three meals per day. If you experience severe hunger between meals, you will allow yourself up to two healthy snacks a day.

There are health benefits to intermittent fasting or time restricted eating (TRE). This involves a daily fast where you only eat only during a certain time span (most often an eight-hour period). This 16-hour daily time without food can be very cleansing for your system and is purported to improve blood sugar, cholesterol and brain function. This form of intermittent fasting often makes it easier for people to decrease total daily caloric intake. You can continue on with this practice if you have found success with it already. If you hadn't tried TRE before and want to try it, start by moving your breakfast ahead or dinner back by one hour and as you adjust, you can slowly widen your fasting window.[13,14,15]

2) *No plans that involve eating less than the TDEE - 500 (or TDEE - 750) numbers.* These plans will slow down your metabolism. Follow too many highly restrictive diets and your body thinks you're back to the cave man era where it may be days until you capture your next meal. Your body does you this wonderful favor of slowing metabolism and storing fat, so you'll stay alive until your next successful hunt. Some restrictive diets have been found to suppress resting metabolic rate (RMR) by as much as 20 percent.[6] They also often lead to mood swings and low energy.

On top of that, if you don't eat enough protein when cutting calories, you may lose muscle mass, which in turn causes further decrease in metabolic rate. That is not a desirable outcome, obviously! Follow that kind of plan and as soon as we start eating normally again, voilà, the weight all piles back on.

Overly restrictive diets leave you hungry and constantly craving everything you shouldn't eat. Please don't make this mistake. Following the *Fitter Than Ever* program should make you feel fabulous, not weak and depressed!

3) *Keep alcohol to a minimum.* Alcohol is nothing but empty calories and can be harmful to more than just the waistline when consumed excessively. I know a geologist who lost 30 pounds in 3 months simply because he was assigned work at a "dry" mining camp (one where no alcohol was allowed). I recommend three drinks or less per week for optimal results.

If you have an alcohol addiction, consider therapy, yoga, and/or meditation. Don't feel like you are alone. Stress can lead people to drink. If you're still working or if you are caring for an aging parent, find more positive ways (exercise, meditation, or a soothing cup of tea, for example) to decompress. Many people drink more after retirement. At first, it might start as a retirement celebration period but then it becomes a permanent habit. Many of the retired people I know abuse alcohol out of boredom, a loss of sense of purpose or to mask depression or physical discomfort.

If you're fit and avoid inflammatory foods (sugar, foods with transfat, and vegetable oils, alcohol, processed meats, foods with monosodium glutamate (MSG), and starchy carbohydrates are the worst culprits), you should experience less age-related physical discomfort.

Filling your day with activities that make you feel useful will ward off depression and reduce the temptation to overindulge in alcohol. You can learn to play a musical instrument, a new language, join an arts and crafts group, or sign up to volunteer in an area of interest. I have found a great deal of fulfillment participating in sea turtle rescue activities with a Mexican marine life rescue group called CRRIFS. I am one of more than 30 volunteers—many of whom are retirees from Mexico, Canada and the United States.

4) *Avoid drinking unnecessary chemicals and calories.* Please avoid sodas, energy drinks, and diet drinks, which contain harmful chemicals and incite hunger due to their high sugar content. Diet drinks are as bad or worse as sugar-laden ones. Aspartame (Nutrasweet, Equal and others) and Sucralose (Splenda and others) have possible links to cancer and neurological disease. [2] Both artificial sweeteners have been

linked to weight gain.[1,3]

Artificial sweeteners are simple carbohydrates that don't provide the body with any nutrients yet cause elevated blood sugar levels. This may increase your desire for and consumption of food and lead to weight gain.

One study found that participants drinking diet soda had a 70 percent greater increase in waist size over a 10-year period compared to non-diet soda drinkers. Those who drank two or more diet sodas a day had a 500 percent greater increase in waist size. Research published in the *Journal of the Academy of Nutrition and Dietetics* indicated that people who drink diet beverages compensate for their "saved" calories by eating more foods high in sugar, sodium and unhealthy fats.[1]

If you drink juice, please consider reducing consumption or switching to water. Most juices have about 120 calories per 8 oz serving. **I know several individuals who have lost up to 10 pounds merely by cutting back on soda and juice. Think about it. Two sodas and two glasses of juice could add up to 500 or 600 calories right there.**

5) *Eliminate mindless eating.* This means no eating in front of your computer, while driving, watching TV or reading. Sit at the table and focus on each bite that enters your mouth! Do you get hungry at night? A good night snack could be a

piece of toast with peanut butter or a cup of grapes or lightly buttered popcorn. I used to drink a cup of warm milk sprinkled with cardamom before bed because it helped me sleep better. Now that I fast 16 hours every day (time restricted eating), I drink chamomile tea before bed instead.

Most people find that food journals unmask a substantial number of calories that previously had slipped by unnoticed.

It will be to your advantage if you avoid eating when you're not hungry. Just because they are serving snacks at a book club group doesn't mean that you have to eat them! Just because food is available doesn't mean you have to eat it. There will be plenty of food around to tempt you tomorrow, the next day and the day after that.

The exception to this rule would be if you are fasting 16 hours daily and are in ketosis often. Fueling your body with fat kills your appetite (a really good thing for many dieters) and so you may need to remind yourself that it's mealtime. If you haven't ever experienced that no hunger feeling, you have something to look forward to!

6) *Chew food well and eat slowly.* Put your fork down often. This will not only improve digestion but will reduce total food consumption. It takes several minutes for your stomach to "register" that it's full.

7) *Pay attention to amount.* If possible, eat on a lunch plate (rather than a large dinner plate) so you are less likely to serve yourself more food than you need to be satisfied. Research has shown people eat less when using smaller plates and plates that have high contrast compared to the color of their food. Meat servings should be no larger than your fist and 75 percent of your plate should be filled with fruits and vegetables. Don't force yourself to finish everything on the plate. Shun seconds unless you are still hungry. If you need to eat more, serve yourself a second helping of broccoli instead of potatoes. You will be less likely to want seconds if you follow rule number 6 above.

8) *Minimize consumption of foods containing MSG,* high fructose corn syrup and low-calorie sweeteners whenever possible. All of these are bad for your health and waistline.

9) *Avoid foods with sugar or high fructose corn syrup.* After the initial "high," your blood sugar will plummet, leaving you feeling tired and hungry. Sugar is an inflammatory food. Sugar shows up in everything, from breakfast cereals to crackers and spaghetti sauce. Read labels – if sugar or high fructose corn syrup sits near the top of the list, don't buy it.

10) *Avoid adding unnecessary calories to food.* You can easily triple or more your calories this way. Avoid fried food, sauces, gravy, and dousing your salad with too much dressing. Consider using a low-cal salad dressing or using olive oil and vinegar instead of high-calorie dressings like Blue Cheese and Thousand Island. Learn to enjoy the flavoring that seasonings provide. Some of my favorites are dill, cinnamon, cardamom, lemon grass, turmeric, basil, garlic, fennel seeds, and oregano. All have very few calories and add wonderful flavor to food. Many are also rich in antioxidants, which reduces inflammation in the body.

11) *Minimize restaurant meals.* It is unlikely you'll lose weight if you eat out more than once or twice a week. In most cases, meals at restaurants tend to be highly caloric, with portions excessively large. You are also forcing yourself to cope with a setting where temptation is everywhere. Choosing a salad will be difficult when your friends are ordering pizza or 16 oz. steaks.

Whenever possible, eat at home where you have control over what's on your plate. Food in your home will be healthier anyway because you can buy good quality organic food rather than eating what the restaurants tend to buy — the cheapest products available.

When you do eat out, go online ahead of time when possible and study the menu so you can decide what to order. Try to steer clear of breadbaskets, chips/salsa and desserts. Make a vow to commit to your healthful choice.

Your meal will be lower in calories if you choose lean meats (fish or chicken, skin removed), broiled, not fried; salads (dressing on the side and light on toppings like bacon and eggs); and meals marked as heart healthy. Opt for a glass of wine or a beer over sugary cocktails and say no to a peek at the dessert menu.

I tend to choose places that serve less caloric foods (sushi bars, Thai or Indian restaurants over pizza places or Mexican restaurants). Avoid all-you-can-eat restaurants like the plague. The food served tends to be packed with fat and calories to save the restaurant money by filling you up, so you won't eat as much. You also could end up eating way past your "full" register simply because (consciously or subconsciously) you think you should "get your money's worth."

12) *Eat 5 to 6 servings of fruits and vegetables daily.* Most fruits and vegetables are low in calories, and many are nutrient-rich. They're also high in fiber and will keep you feeling full longer. If you're craving sweet and delicious fruits, try mangoes and papayas. I'd rather have those than cookies!

13) *Choose carbohydrates wisely.* Whole grain bread over white, whole grain pasta over white, wild rice over white, organic oatmeal over cold cereals laden with sugar and preservatives. These high-fiber choices will also improve digestion and give you a sense of fullness that will last for hours.

Most "starchy" carbohydrates such as white bread, pies, cookies, cakes and crackers are loaded with fat and preservatives and provide little in the way of vitamins and minerals. These simple carbohydrates quickly assault your blood stream, raising blood sugar for a short period of time before you experience another sugar crash.

People who eat a lot of starchy carbohydrates tend to reflexively reach for more sugar whenever they experience a sugar crash. This is a vicious cycle that needs to be broken. Don't fall in the trap of buying junk that is labeled "low-fat" or "organic." If it's got a list of ingredients a mile long, you don't want to buy it. I rarely buy anything with more than three or four ingredients.

Try to start replacing starchy carbohydrates with complex carbohydrates (whole grains). Oatmeal, whole grain breads, quinoa, and wild rice are some examples of complex carbohydrates.

If you're gluten intolerant, suffer from migraines, or have other digestive issues, you may want to eliminate grains from your diet. I have been following this protocol for almost three years now.

14) *Have a glass of water before you eat.* You will feel full sooner just by drinking the water.

15) *Avoid arriving to parties hungry.* Have a light snack before you leave the house. When you arrive, fill a small plate once and step away from the serving table to talk. Slowly eat what's on your plate and then discard it so you're not tempted to graze later on.

16) *Drink a small recovery drink* after any high intensity or long-duration (more than an hour) workout, preferably something with fat, carbohydrates, and protein. Four ounces of low-fat chocolate milk (94 calories) is a good choice. My husband makes his own in a blender with cocoa to avoid the sugar.

17) *Eliminate emotional eating.* This is tricky for many of us. Most of us choose to eat more or less because of emotions. Some of us overeat when upset while others shun food when suffering. If you find that you tend to use food to soothe

emotions and you want to lose weight, it will serve you well to work to replace this habit with another behavior.

I actually succeeded at this toward the end of my college days. Throughout high school and college, whenever I was upset, I would binge eat. But it never made me feel better. In fact, it made me feel much worse. I felt bloated and drowsy and guilty.

So, I decided to start exercising whenever I was upset. Okay, so maybe I would overdo it a little. I would go out and run until my legs threatened to give out underneath me. Was that extreme? Yes. But it made me feel empowered. I've found writing to be another powerful outlet for stress and suffering. To this day, I tend to exercise, meditate, or write over grabbing a bag of chips whenever stress strikes. And there are no negative side effects either (weight gain, guilt, poor health).

We're all wired differently so maybe you won't find exercise or writing to be the right activities to replace your emotional eating. Use whatever feeds your soul—so that you'll feel better afterward. Other positive indulgences could be a conversation with a friend, time outdoors in a quiet park, a warm bath (with bubbles or nice smelling salts), playing a musical instrument, painting or drawing, getting a massage or pedicure, or reading. All of these are likely to release "feel good" hormones and won't leave you with a guilt hangover.

18) *If you get off track, jump back on instead of continuing to binge or eat the wrong foods.* Remember, you have to eat an excess of 3500 calories to gain a pound, so if you slip up and eat two pieces of pie one night, you won't gain weight as long as you avoid overeating the rest of the day. Forgive and forget, rather than allowing yourself to tumble into the abyss of guilt and recrimination. If you get back on track quickly, you'll keep losing weight.

Keep in mind that these changes may be challenging for a while but should become part of your lifestyle by the end of this trial. Once healthy eating becomes a habit, adhering will no longer be difficult.

4) The Tracking Plan

You will find it helpful to collect baseline information. By knowing where you stand today, it will be easier to determine where you want to go. Watching changes will be exciting and help inspire you to keep going.

1 - Measure circumference of the following and record in your journal:

Chest (across the nipples)

Hips

Waist

Right Thigh (at widest part)

Left Thigh (at widest part)

Right arm (at widest part)

Left arm (at widest part)

Calf (at widest part)

Re-measure and record every 30 days.

2 - Measure and Record Body Fat Percentage or Calculated BMI and Ideal Bodyweight (from Table below).

The terms Body Fat Percentage and Body Mass Index (BMI) are probably familiar to you. The Body Fat Percentage is the percentage of fat on your body compared to your fat-free mass (blood, bones, muscles, organs, etc). Knowing this number allows you to most accurately calculate your ideal weight. If you want to know your body fat percentage, you can have this measured at most fitness facilities. Many personal trainers will do skin caliper tests or use bioelectrical impedance equipment to compute these numbers for you and both of these methods are fairly accurate. Otherwise, you can use the table below to determine your BMI.

Body Mass Index (BMI) is an estimate of your body fat percentage based exclusively on your height and weight. You can work with a BMI number instead of body fat percentage if it's more convenient for you. These numbers can sometimes be misleading for individuals with either high or low amounts of muscle. You can go to the U.S. Health and Human Services website and enter your height and weight to obtain your BMI - https://www.nhlbi.nih.gov/health/educational/lose_wt/BMI/bmicalc.htm

The American College of Sports Medicine has established the following norms for BMI for adult women and men.

Underweight < 18.5

Normal 18.5-24.9

Overweight 25-29.9

Obese 30.0-39.9

Extreme Obesity > 40.0

Table 1. BMI Chart to Estimate Ideal Weight [10]

Body Weight in Pounds According to Height and Body Mass Index													
BMI (kg/m2)	19	20	21	22	23	24	25	26	27	28	29	30	35	40
Ht (in)	Weight (lbs.)													
58	91	96	100	105	110	115	119	124	129	134	138	143	167	191
59	94	99	104	109	114	119	124	128	133	138	143	148	173	198
60	97	102	107	112	118	123	128	133	138	143	148	153	179	204
61	100	106	111	116	122	127	132	137	143	148	153	158	185	211
62	104	109	115	120	126	131	136	142	147	153	158	164	191	218
63	107	113	118	124	130	135	141	146	152	158	163	169	197	225
64	110	116	122	128	134	140	145	151	157	163	169	174	204	232
65	114	120	126	132	138	144	150	156	162	168	174	180	210	240
66	118	124	130	136	142	148	155	161	167	173	179	186	216	247
67	121	127	134	140	146	153	159	166	172	178	185	191	223	255
68	125	131	138	144	151	158	164	171	177	184	190	197	230	262
69	128	135	142	149	155	162	169	176	182	189	196	203	236	270
70	132	139	146	153	160	167	174	181	188	195	202	207	243	278
71	136	143	150	157	165	172	179	186	193	200	208	215	250	286
72	140	147	154	162	169	177	184	191	199	206	213	221	258	294
73	144	151	159	166	174	182	189	197	204	212	219	227	265	302
74	148	155	163	171	179	186	194	202	210	218	225	233	272	311
75	152	160	168	176	184	192	200	208	216	224	232	240	279	319
76	156	164	172	180	189	197	205	213	221	230	238	246	287	328

Table 2. Personal Record of BMI or Body Fat Percent

Date			
BMI			
BF %			

Construct a table similar to the one above in your journal. Record your BMI and the date. Measure BMI every three months so you can track your improvement and stay inspired. Weigh yourself in the early morning. Record your weight in your journal once a week (always on the same day) in a chart similar to Table 3.

It is normal to hit a plateau while you're losing weight. Try not to let this discourage you. Most people who persist with their computed weight loss caloric intake and regular exercise break through it within a few days. If your plateau continues for more than two weeks, increase exercise and reduce daily intake by 200 calories. Make sure you measure quantities accurately and that no hidden calories (mayonnaise, sauces, gravy, etc.) slip past your radar.

3 - Construct a table similar to the one below in your journal. Record the number of pounds you want to lose (current weight minus desired weight). Continue to track weight on the same day and time each week.

Table 3. Chart for Weekly Weight & Weight Loss Goal

Date	Current Weight	Desired Weight (from BMI Chart or Goals)	Pounds to Lose (CW-DW)

4 - Continue with your food journal as explained in the previous section.

5 - Track your daily exercise. Record the date, modality of

exercise, intensity, and total number of minutes. It can also be helpful to record some notes about how you felt during and after your workouts and which kinds of exercise you enjoyed the most.

5) The Lifestyle Plan. I've already mentioned this, but the main objective of this program is reprogramming how you live so regular exercise and healthy eating become as routine as brushing your teeth. Until these become habits it is very important for you to record your daily and weekly exercise and eating so you can chart your progress. Record what is working for you and what is getting in the way pertaining to both the exercise and the nutritional components and begin to devise strategies that help you to get through the bumps in your road to success.

Below are some suggestions for overcoming problem habits:

Skipping workouts – Start attending group classes or enlist support from a friend. Block out specific times for exercise each week and enter them in your smartphone or computer calendar. Set an alarm on your smartphone for an hour before you plan to exercise to remind you.

Stress eating – Substitute a healthy activity for overeating that will more effectively release your stress such as exercise, a warm bath, massage, listening to relaxing music, meditation, reading, or visiting with a friend. There are many free Yoga Nidra meditations for stress and anxiety you can listen to free on YouTube or you can download the Insight Timer or other apps on your device.

Night eating – if you crave an evening snack, try a glass of warm milk, which will relax you, help you sleep and give you a sense of fullness. If you're accustomed to eating dinner late, slowly move your mealtime to an earlier time if possible. Going to bed on a full stomach may cause indigestion and impair quality sleep.

Mindless eating – Just say no...Any food you eat when distracted won't satisfy you and you'll end up feeling hungry or craving food again soon. Put down your fork between bits and notice every bite that goes in your mouth.

Excessive Alcohol Consumption – If your alcohol consumption is destroying your health and relationships, seek help through Alcoholics Anonymous or get counseling. If you drink to reduce stress, start to replace the drinking with a healthy behavior as mentioned above. Aim to cut back to no more than two or three drinks per week. It is best to quit altogether, of course, if you have an addiction.

I completely stopped drinking a few years ago because even one drink would interfere with sleep, cause headache, or leave me feeling very lethargic the next day (which is rare for me because I usually have a lot of energy).

6) **The Motivation Plan.** Participate in activities such as walkathons, triathlons, cycling group rides, etc. to keep motivation high. If at all possible, find a friend or spouse to join you. If you choose a competitive event, track your time in your journal, so you can chart your progress if you do the same event or a similar distance race again.

At least once a month, sign up for some kind of "athletic" event. It can be a 5K walk/run, a triathlon or a walkathon for your favorite cause. If you have never done a group event, please don't be intimidated. Most people who sign up for these events are not stellar athletes. Most participants are people who want to get out there and do something healthy and mingle and socialize with other people who care about their health. Once you find out how fun these events can be, you will look forward to the next one.

7) The Susan's Slim for Life Secrets Plan

At the end of this book, I have listed more than 20 Slim for Life Secrets that have enabled me to stay fit while many people my age have gained weight and lost conditioning. These tips can give you that extra edge you need to succeed.

I hope you're pumped up about this journey to wellness! These key lifestyle changes will leave you feeling better than ever before and you won't believe how good it feels when people come up and say, "You look amazing." It's about to happen to you. Believe you can do it, work hard, and you will succeed.

REFERENCES

1 - An, R. 2016. "Beverage Consumption in Relation to Discretionary Food Intake and Diet Quality among US Adults, 2003 to 2012." *Journal of the Academy of Nutrition and Dietetics*. 116(1):28-37.

2 - Comana, F. 2012. The Energy Balance Equation. *IDEA Fitness Journal*. 9(3).

3 - Center for Science in the Public Interest. 2013. "CSPI Downgrades Splenda from 'Safe' to 'Caution.'" https://cspinet.org/new/201306121.html

4 - Ford, H.E., V. Peters, N.M. Martin, M.L. Sleeth, M.A. Ghatei, G.S. Frost, and S.R. Bloom. 2011. "Effects of oral ingestion of sucralose on gut hormone response and appetite in healthy normal-weight subjects." *European Journal of Clinical Nutrition*. 65 (4): 508–13.

5 - Grattan, B.J., Jr., and J. Connolly-Schoonen, J. 2012. "Addressing weight loss recidivism: a clinical focus on metabolic rate and the psychological aspects of obesity." *ISRN Obesity*. 2012: 567530.

6 - Hill, A.J. 2004. "Does dieting make you fat?" *British Journal of Nutrition, 92*(1), S5–S18.

7 - Manini, T.M. 2010. "Energy expenditure and aging." *Ageing Research Reviews.* 9(1): 1-11.

8 - Matthews, M. Muscle for Life
https://www.muscleforlife.com/tdee-calculator/

9 - McMurray, R.G., J. Soares, C.J. Casperson, C.J, and T. McCurdy. 2014. "Examining variations of resting metabolic rate of adults: a public health perspective." *Medicine and Sciences in Sports and Exercise.* 46 (7): 1352-1358.

10 - National Heart, Blood, and Lung Institute
https://www.nhlbi.nih.gov/health/educational/lose_wt/BMI/bmi_tbl.htm

11 - Hall, J., S.M. Skevington, P.J. Maddison, and K. Chapman. 1996. "A randomized and controlled trial of hydrotherapy in rheumatoid arthritis." *Arthritis Care Research*, 9(3): 206-215.

12- Wyatt, F.B., S. Milam, R.C. Manske, and R. Deere. 2001. "The effects of aquatic and traditional exercise programs on persons with knee osteoarthritis," *Journal of Strength Conditioning Research*, 15(3): 337-340.

13 – Chow, L., E. Manoogian, A. Alvear, J. Fleischer, H. Thor, K. Dietsche, Q. Wang, J. Hodges, N. Esch, S. Malaeb, T. Harindhanavudhi, K. Nair, S. Panda, and D. Mashek. 2020. "Time Restricted Eating Effects on Body Composition and Metabolic Measures in Humans Who are Overweight: A Feasibility Study." *Obesity.* 28(5): 860-869.

14 - Wilkinson M., E. Manoogian, A. Zadourian, H. Lo, S. Fakhouri, A. Shoghi, X. Wang, J. Fleisher, S Navlakha, S.

Panda, and P. Taub. 2020. "Ten-Hour Time-Restricted Eating Reduces Weight, Blood Pressure, and Atherogenic Lipids in Patients with Metabolic Syndrome." *Cell Metabolism* 31(1): 92–104.e105.

15 - Sutton E.F., R. Beyl, K.S. Early, W.T. Cefalu, E. Ravussin, and C.M. Peterson. 2018. "Early Time-Restricted Feeding Improves Insulin Sensitivity, Blood Pressure, and Oxidative Stress Even without Weight Loss in Men with Prediabetes." *Cell Metabolism* 27(6): 1212–1221.e3.

16 – McArdle, W., R. Glasner, and J. Magel. 1971. "Metabolic and cardio-respiratory responses during free swimming and treadmill walking." *Journal of Applied Physiology*. 33(5): 733-738.

CHAPTER TWO

A Day in the Life of Susan (from age 17 to 24)

My major weight struggles started when I was 17. I was a competitive swimmer, a junior in high school and had started to experience weight gain anytime I was in the off-season. Sometimes I'd pack on more than ten pounds over the course of a month-long break.

People began to comment. One of my assistant coaches, Bob, told one of my teammates, "Susan's getting fat." At first, I heard the word "fast" and was shattered when I found out he'd actually said "fat." I wanted my coaches to see me as an athlete with promise, not this.

My private school headmaster, Mr. Chapman, said I was too fat to be an athlete. I really resented his comment since he was what would be considered obese, while I was maybe 10 pounds over my ideal weight and only when not training.

My brother also criticized my body, but my father's comments hurt the most. He would monitor my eating and tell me I shouldn't eat this or that. He would buy doughnuts and potato chips and he would eat them whenever he wanted, but he always threw out a cutting comment if I ate any.

It angered me because he wasn't thin or even in very good shape. I didn't understand why if he had a belly and I was barely overweight according to height/weight charts, why I deserved to suffer this deluge of criticism. It felt unfair. And all the emotional turmoil this caused me made me want to eat more than ever.

So, I started hiding junk food under my bed. I'd eat chips and doughnuts when no one was looking. If no one saw me, eating was safe.

I attended an all-girls, college-prep school and swam three hours almost daily. After studying and training I didn't have much time for socializing. I rarely had a date.

Because my body leaned toward muscular when trained hard, many of the guys on my team called me names that made me feel unfeminine and unattractive, like "Muscles Mahoney" and "Flex Armstrong." I started to suspect the extra weight and my large muscular arms were a turn off to guys. I didn't look anything like the women on the magazine covers or that graced the posters my dad had posted in his office closet. They had spaghetti arms and no apparent muscle; I had broad (size 12) shoulders and triceps that bulged and flexed.

I started reading fitness and teen magazines that focused on diet and weight. I embarked on countless fad diets and even made myself vomit occasionally. By the time I graduated from high school, I had a full-blown eating disorder.

I was depressed, suffered from food phobia, vomited up meals fairly often and popped diet pills to try to tamp down my appetite. At night, I dreamed about food. My entire life became a vicious cycle of eating, not eating, and thinking about food and dieting. When my body didn't reshape the way I wished it would or someone criticized my appearance, I often felt like I would drown in self-loathing.

Things only worsened when I graduated from high school and went to Clemson University. When I quit competitive swimming my sophomore year, I gained weight almost immediately. I stopped purging because it left me feeling guilty and wreaked havoc on my self-esteem, not to mention my health. But I continued to try fad diets and to fight my body, instead of seeking a way to establish harmony with it. I still craved the same food quantity I had consumed when training hard even though my body no longer needed that many calories. Drinking alcohol and ordering pizzas late at night after parties didn't help either. I was using alcohol and food as crutches to console my feelings of despair and inadequacy. By the time I graduated, I had packed on 30 pounds.

For too long, I denied I had a problem. I wore loose clothes and forced myself to do exercise I hated. Was I frustrated? Yes, I felt very discouraged and bad about myself. I had 2 AM cravings for pizza and all the other snack foods I kept in my dorm room. After one or more drinks out with my friends, my discipline would be out the window and I'd drink until I was intoxicated and then eat whatever kind of junk food I craved the rest of the night.

I started to hate exercise. I found lap swimming monotonous. I was used to the camaraderie of a team and laughing and joking with friends between sets. I would slog out the miles in the pool alone and feel miserable. I sometimes ran and only found it enjoyable on the rare occasion I found someone to join me. It wasn't a big shocker people weren't lining up to run with me. Pounding out miles in the heat and humidity of South Carolina was sheer misery.

Because of a relationship, I stayed in Clemson for two years after graduating. One day I went to the student recreation center with my swimming gear, prepared to slog out another hour of boring laps. Suddenly, I heard music from the gymnasium. I walked down the hall and saw more than 50 people were following the athletic dance moves of a college girl in tights and a thong leotard. Students and faculty—men and women alike—with varying degrees of physical coordination, attempted to emulate her well-choreographed routine.

That looks like fun, I thought. There was so much energy in the room, and everyone was smiling and looking more like they were dancing to music at a nightclub than doing a workout. The music was energetic and made me want to jump around myself. I'd inadvertently walked into the right place at the right time. I had found exercise that looked fun in a setting with the social aspect I sought.

In no time, I was taking classes 5 days a week (I even rushed out and bought some colorful leotards and—it was the 80s—a few pairs of leg warmers). Now that I had gotten my butt moving, I would whip my diet into shape, I told myself.

I checked out books on nutrition from the library and started to build my diet around nutritional food. I cut back to less than 5 drinks per week (today, I don't drink at all), prepared healthy meals that I didn't find appetizing at first. I had to learn all over to appreciate the taste of healthy food (my mother fed me very healthy meals and snacks when I was a youth—how quickly I forgot).

I didn't want to "diet" anymore. I wanted to be healthy for the sake of my own desires and objectives, not struggle to fit an image that my father or my boyfriend du jour had of the ideal body shape. I embarked on a mission to live healthier, which led to many discoveries, including a fitness instructor certification and eventually a career in fitness.

The weight didn't melt off overnight, but it came off pound by pound. Over the course of five years, my body transformed from broad shouldered and bulky to lean and defined.

My disordered eating vanished when I stopped trying to "diet," fit into other peoples' concepts of "thin," and instead focused on wellness. I stopped forcing myself to miss meals and ditched the junk food and chose activities for the sake of enjoyment rather than for the sake of "burning off" what I'd just eaten.

I followed my new healthy lifestyle program because I wanted to, not because someone said I should. If you change your habits for the sake of *your* health and *your* well being, not to satisfy the male image of the ideal woman or because your husband says your fanny jiggles, you have a much higher chance of succeeding.

From experience I can say you won't be having the time of your life every day you're following this program. At times, you'll want to quit. You may even want to yell at me.

Tell me you would rather have a root canal than stick with this program. It's very hard to break bad habits. For years, many of your lives have involved too much eating, too much self-recrimination, and too little exercise.

What at first will be painful will in the end be the best thing you've ever done for yourself! If you keep your eye on your long-term goals and notice the small positive changes, you'll not only succeed, you'll feel happy and empowered in the process.

You'll have more energy. You'll probably sleep much better. You'll feel less irritable when your spouse leaves the garage door open. Your pants will start fitting looser. Friends will at first say you look great and then will remark that you look thinner. Each little burst of progress can fuel your desire to keep going.

Since I traveled down the wrong road and came back again, I can honestly make some declarations to you. You don't have to carry around a 20-pound spare tire around your middle just because many of your contemporaries do.

You don't have to follow fad diets, starve yourself or pop pills to lose weight and start living in a trimmer body. The decision is yours. I'm giving you all the tools you need to succeed. Will you convince yourself that a fit physique at "your age" is impossible and set yourself up for failure before you even start? Or will you get psyched and embark on this *Fitter Than Ever* program that will leave you feeling better than ever?

CHAPTER THREE

A Day in the Life of Susan (Today)

Since the publication of *Fitter Than Ever at 40 and Beyond*, I retired from full-time work and now live most of the year in San Carlos, Mexico. Although I ate very healthy before, I changed my diet three years ago to improve my digestion and blood sugar levels. I think it is very important to pay attention to how your body reacts to certain foods and make adjustments that work best for your health as needed.

I used to eat healthy snacks all day—now I eat only three times a day—never snacking and fast 15 or more hours daily, so my body is sometimes in ketosis (relying on body fat instead of available sugar from food for energy). I also have eliminated grains, sugar, and alcohol from my diet.

These dietary shifts are not required as part of the *Fitter Than Ever* plan but there are some big benefits to this way of eating, which I'll share with you. What I love most about eating like this is that I have almost no digestive issues and I never experience extreme hunger because my body has learned to be versatile and now shifts easily from using food for energy to using fat for energy.

I consume more fat than I used to, emphasizing healthy fats, such as is found in avocados and olive oil. Foods with higher fat content tend to contain a lot of nutrients your body needs, take longer for your body to burn, and keep you feeling full longer. Many carbohydrate-rich foods, on the other hand, tend to be nutrient-poor and often contribute to unwieldy hunger.

Since I don't get hungry as often (or at all, most of the time), I can go longer periods of time without food and so I don't have to pack snacks with me wherever I go or worry as much about food when traveling. For dieters, this is an amazing benefit because you kiss horrible, painful, gnawing hunger goodbye for good, which makes reducing caloric intake easy. Having control over your hunger and food consumption can be very empowering.

If you do decide to go gluten and sugar free, make sure you track food consumption for long enough to determine how to obtain a good nutritional balance from the foods you're eating.

Most days, my husband and I get up about 5 AM. We drink a cup of coffee together and then walk our Chow

Chow, Chief, about an hour later. Then I change into my swimsuit and head down to the beach for my hour-long sea swim. Occasionally, I cross train with running or hiking.

I eat breakfast between 9 and 10 AM. My breakfast normally consists of a tablespoon of melted butter, a cup of homemade organic yogurt topped with a variety of fruit (blueberries, papaya, raspberries, grapes, and/or strawberries) and nuts (pecans, macadamia nuts, or walnuts, usually).

During the day, I write, teach yoga classes, volunteer with a Mexican marine life rescue group, and shop. Now that I'm not working full-time, I sometimes enjoy long lunches with friends or sit on the beach under our tent and read.

For lunch (around 1 or 2 PM), I often eat a scrambled or hard-boiled egg, four cherry tomatoes, 12 almonds, about a half a cup of potato chips (only potatoes, olive oil and salt), three or four slices of cheese and a half of an avocado. Sometimes I have canned salmon or bonita (a fish my neighbor catches often and cans) instead of an egg.

For dinner, we usually have a serving of meat with a very large salad or serving of vegetables. I really enjoy a tasty ribeye!

Before or after dinner, we take Chief out for another walk and spend our evenings watching the sunset at the beach or reading usually. I have a cup of chamomile tea about a half hour before going to bed. We call it a night early usually — usually between 8:30 and 9:30 PM.

CHAPTER FOUR

Retirement Can Enhance or Deep-Six Wellness

Many people in their 50s reach the pinnacle of their careers, acquiring their ideal professional positions and levels of earning they've always wanted. Women often have more time to dedicate to their careers, with children reaching adulthood or leaving the nest. For those of you who are still busy working professionals, you can skip this chapter for now and refer back to it when you are ready to plan for retirement.

Those of you who are currently retired or planning to retire soon can use this chapter as a guide to help you improve your diet and exercise habits instead of losing ground during this phase of your lives. The choices you make during this critical stage will be key to your future physical and mental health and quality of life for years to come.

I will begin by sharing my recent retirement experiences and then move on to sharing what research studies show is common for retirees to experience when it comes to exercise and dietary habits.

I retired from full-time work in my mid-50s and found on the whole the experience to be a tremendous blessing. I've always dreamed of living by a sea or ocean where I could hear the sound of crashing waves and swim whenever I wanted.

This dream came true when we bought a seaside condo in San Carlos, Mexico and started living down there most of the year. The expatriate lifestyle is one of many benefits to me of retiring. The reduced cost of living here—and the simplification of our standards for what we "need"—enabled us to retire earlier than we originally planned without jeopardizing our financial future.

Throughout my working years, I always maintained a high activity level regardless of my work schedule (even when traveling 50 or more percent of the time). High levels of activity benefitted my work performance, enhancing mental focus and energy level, and keeping stress at bay.

My "retirement" has been a transition from full-time work to very part-time work, enhanced with volunteer activities. I now teach several yoga classes weekly, pursue professional and "just for fun" writing projects, and support a sea turtle rescue volunteer effort in San Carlos. This has been a very positive choice for my mental health. Keeping busy helps me feel like I'm contributing, keeps me connected to my community, and helps me stay mentally sharp.

Having more free time has enabled me to spend more time with friends and family, volunteer, read, play the violin, and practice Spanish. I even occasionally take an art class at a local shop and try my hand at making candles or windchimes!

I can now exercise without rushing and grabbing meals on the run. If I happen to run into the friendly pod of bottlenose dolphins during my morning sea swims, I can stop and visit with them or to just float on my back and soak up the view of the dramatic volcanic landscape and passing clouds from the blue-green water. This slower-paced life really suits me.

Practicing yoga in recent years has been transformative for me during this phase of my life. Many people feel inadequate and insignificant after they retire. Mindful practice has shifted my mental frame-of-reference from a traditional view of success to a more spiritually-based value system.

I knew that I needed to make this change five years ago when I decided to get my RYT-200 Yoga Alliance certification. I didn't want to take a weekend class and drift in and out of a yogic lifestyle. I wanted to immerse myself in mindful living. Weeks later, I flew to Big Corn Island, Nicaragua for a three-week yoga teacher training. Big Corn is a remote island in the Caribbean, what many travelers have dubbed "Gilligan's Island."

When I was shown my small dark room, roofed in palm fronds, I looked around and swore to myself that I couldn't sleep on that mattress on a cement platform, shower under a stream of cold water, and get by in such a small, dreary space for three whole weeks. I lived in a large, beautiful house in Oro Valley, Arizona with travertine floors and a pool and spa in the backyard. I deserved better than this, I told myself.

Three days later, I noticed that I felt more joy and contentment than I'd ever experienced in my entire life and began to question my previous dissatisfaction with my small room. The serene, happy feelings I had weren't linked to physical comfort or any material possessions, they were linked to feelings of connection — with nature, with the other people in my yoga training, with myself.

I had awoken each morning at 5 AM, walked down a shell-lined path to the beach to enjoy a swim in the Caribbean Sea. I saw schools of spotted rays flapping their way gracefully through the crystal-clear water, schools of blue tangs and pairs of orange and black angel fish nibbling on plants on a spectacular, multi-colored coral reef. And a nurse shark resting, just visible below a ledge of coral.

All day, as I learned and practiced yoga, I heard birds singing, felt the alternating breath of sea air and the scorching humidity of Nicaragua's summer heat on my skin. During our early evening practice, I heard laughing children on a nearby field playing soccer. I became a part of this remote, Nicaraguan island. It became a sanctuary.

Experiencing the beauty of nature and interacting harmoniously with it and enjoying meaningful interactions with the yogis in my class—this was living. The block and thatch structure where I studied and slept seemed much more than adequate. Lasting happiness, I knew then, could never come from a fancy house, a new car, or a designer dress. Day by day, material possessions began to lose importance.

Years earlier, the efforts we went through to buy our big fancy house (a short sale) in Tucson had become all encompassing—acquiring that house felt like the most important thing in the world. I believed once we owned that house, my life would be so much better. It now seemed silly that I had placed so much importance on owning a material object. The house was beautiful, but it hadn't delivered the happiness I expected. In a way, owning the house had detracted from our happiness—saddling us with debt, little money to travel, and many maintenance headaches.

Soon after returning from the yoga teacher training, I told my husband I wanted a different life. After researching possible beach residences in Panama, Costa Rica, and Mexico, we decided to buy a property in San Carlos, Mexico—a day's drive from Tucson—and to sell the large and expensive (for us) Tucson house, replacing it with a simpler place.

We now own a small, seaside condo in Mexico and a small, easy care house in a tranquil Tucson neighborhood. We are free of all mortgage and debt, which provides us an amazing sense of freedom.

Helping a neighbor in need or supporting my marine rescue group feels much more like success today than big earnings, impressive book sales figures, or fancy job titles. I'm honestly very content with who I am and feel successful any day I experience personal growth and contribute in some positive way to others (humans or other creatures we share this earth with).

People who practice yoga regularly often experience a mental shift because calming the mind with the breath enables one to filter out the clutter of erratic thoughts, news reports, and other peoples' expectations and standards, which enables better self-understanding. Once you know what really matters to you, where your true values lie, the pathway to happiness is much more straightforward.

Another benefit of mindful practices such as yoga, meditation and Yoga Nidra is that they can tamp down anxiety and depression. Many people suffer from age-associated anxiety and depression. These practices can help to bring your mind and body back into a state of harmony and balance.

Research has shown that retirement creates significant shifts in diet, exercise, and body weight. Interestingly enough, people tend to make a shift in either a positive or negative health direction post-retirement. You have the opportunity to use retirement to your advantage so you can be fitter and slimmer than you were while working. Let's discuss the good, the bad and the ugly when it comes to retirement, diet, exercise, and lifestyle choices.

First for the good news. Many retired Masters swimmers I know have upped the ante on their training now that they have more time. Instead of training for 100 or 200-yard pool swimming races, they're training for 5 K open water swims or triathlons, often spending two or more hours swimming or training daily. In case you're not familiar with U.S. Masters swimming—it's a national swimming program for adults where swimmers have the opportunity to work out with a team and participate in local and national competition if they choose to do so. You can join, read articles and see the schedule of competitions and more at usms.org. The camaraderie of having people to train and race with can be so much fun.

Many friends in my swimming and yoga community travel more due to their new-found freedom. And often the trips they choose include activity — cycling trips in Europe, open water swimming trips, hikes to the tops of volcanoes and to ancient ruins and more.

One Mexican couple we know in their 70s hike the Camino de Santiago in Europe almost every summer. So many people we know are using their newly found freedom to enhance their health by keeping active. And their training sessions, competitions, and trips with others provide them with fun experiences, opportunities to meet new friends, and memories that last a lifetime.

As a retiree, you can no longer can use that worn out excuse that there isn't enough time to exercise. You have plenty of time now to swim, walk, jog, or take an exercise class. You have plenty of time to try different modalities to discover what kind of exercise you enjoy most and that agrees with your body. You also are at that stage where if you aren't currently exercising, inertia will lure you to continue on with this unhealthy, sedentary way of living. It is important to kick off this new phase of your life with plenty of activity so you can move in the direction of wellness.

As a retiree, you have more choices about what you eat. You're no longer required to attend lunch meetings or take work-related trips, where restaurant meals are your only option. During his years working as an IT manager, my husband constantly complained about meals ordered in for meetings. He'd come home from work, wanting to skip dinner because he still felt stuffed from lunch. Instead of the healthy salads and simple sandwiches he preferred as lunch foods, the company tended to order catered meals that featured fattening foods with heavy sauces like ribs, pizzas and pasta dishes.

As a retiree, you now have total control over food buying, food preparation, and food consumption. Your mission—should you choose to accept it—is to use this freedom to your advantage.

Many retirees have the option of living wherever they choose. If the climate where you currently live isn't what you like (or isn't conducive for daily exercise), you can pack up and move to a seaside cottage or a cabin in the mountains. Millions of retirees like my husband and I have embarked on the expatriate life—moving to another country for a new adventure. Many of our friends spend winters in Mexico and the rest of the year in Canada or the US.

Now it's time to share the bad news. Having trained hundreds of recently retired clients, I know that many of them faced obstacles post-retirement. Some found themselves feeling bored and depressed when not working. They had identified so strongly with that job title they once held, they no longer felt useful. This stagnant state of existence often led them to heavy drinking and using food for solace.

Others turned their focus from work to a constant obsession with health and the possibility of sickness. They constantly worried they had acquired this disease or that disorder and often cancelled training appointments for unnecessary visits to their physicians and other specialists.

Many clients complained about food and drink being served at literally every social event. Almost every day there was a dinner at a neighbor's or an HOA meeting (with cookies), or a book club meeting (with chips and nuts and a bottle or two of wine on the side). With food as a constant temptation, many felt that weight gain was unavoidable and that shunning food that was offered would make them unpopular with friends and neighbors.

A French study of more than 12,000 participants showed an increase of saturated fatty acids and sodium ingested post-retirement. Women ate fewer fruits and more sweets. Men tended to eat more foods higher in fats.

Overall, retired men tended to adopt the worst post-retirement dietary practices. [2]

This study is significant because following healthy dietary guidelines is critical to disease management. Unhealthy eating predisposes people to cardiovascular illness, type 2 diabetes, cancer, hypertension and a host of other illnesses. Is the discomfort over declining a dessert or a serving of snacks worth the health consequences? It isn't to me!

I've learned to say "no" when offered food I don't want. I do it politely, but I don't cave in under pressure. Yes, people will say, "Can't you eat dessert just this once?" or "You should live a little," but often they are putting this pressure on you because they don't have the discipline to make healthy food choices. So, I encourage you not to give in. After a while, you'll find your ability to stand your ground very empowering.

You can kindly decline to eat the nuts, cookies, chips and other (usually unhealthy or highly caloric foods) being offered at your book club or association meeting. Another option is to host events and to simply serve drinks if it is not during a mealtime. It may be an adjustment for people at first, but in the long run, most of your friends will be grateful to be able to enjoy the company of friends sometimes without the temptation of food around.

Retirees have reported loss of status, identity, purpose, and the social support they had at their workplaces as reasons for life dissatisfaction post-retirement. Many resort to increased alcohol consumption or even alcohol abuse as a result.

A recent study in *Alcoholism: Clinical and Experimental Research*, based on a survey of 65,303 women over 60 showed an increase of binge drinking by 3.7 percent per year. A significant increase in alcohol consumption can lead to weight gain and a variety of health problems. [3]

Women are more likely than men to gain weight after retirement. Cited in the research as reasons for post-retirement weight gain are reduced physical activity, less-structured meal times, and eating in response to loss of personal identity or the potential for social interactions. Women retirees averaged a five percent weight gain over a period of two years. [1]

But this same research study determined that some individuals actually lost weight post-retirement when work-related meals out were no longer required and more time for exercise was available.

You have the option to choose wisely — so retirement tips the scale in a downward rather than an upward direction due to wise choices. Make a commitment to eat healthier and increase your activity level as you transition into these golden years.

REFERENCES

1 - Forman-Hoffman, V., K. Richardson, J. Yankey, S. Hillis, R. Wallace, and F. Wolinsky. 2008. "Retirement and Weight Changes Amon Men and Women in the Health and Retirement Study." *The Journals of Gerontology*. 63(3): S146-S153.

2 - Lauque, S., F. Nourashemi, C. Soleilhavoup, S. Guyonnet, M.C. Bertiere, P. Sachet, B. Vellas, and J.L. Albarede. 1998. "A prospective study of changes on nutritional patterns 6 months before and 18 months after retirement. *Journal of Nutrition, Health, and Aging*. 2(2): 88-91.

3 – Breslow, R., I.J. Castle, C. Chjung; and B. Graubard. 2017. "Trends in Alcohol Consumption Among Older Americans: National Health Interview Surveys, 1997-2014." *Alcohol Clin Exp Res*. 41(5): 976-986.

CHAPTER FIVE

Does Menopause Make You Fat?

I lost count of the number of overweight female clients who swear they were "super thin" until menopause and then "all of a sudden" gained 20, 30 or even 50 pounds. When I first started training clients 14 years ago, I was stymied (and a little scared). I was 42 at the time and wondered…Could that happen to me?

At that time, I had survived the birth of my two children and turning 40 without weight gain even though in the past I had heard "wait until you have children" and then "after your second child, you'll gain weight and never be able to get it off." Then people began to say, "after menopause strikes, that trim waist of yours will disappear" or something similar.

Menopause loomed and a nagging voice in my head made me wonder if my female transition would mark doomsday for my flat stomach. But then I told myself I'd heard similar doomsday weight gain warnings in the past, and none had come to fruition. Even before menopause, I had begun to suspect that the shape you have is much more the result of your life habits and your attitude than childbirth or any other phase of life.

Fortunately for me, I had already taught myself how to eat and exercise right and told myself I had nothing to fear from menopause or any other transition. I'm now 58 and still haven't gained a single pound.

I've read numerous articles suggesting that fluctuating and dropping hormones could result in body changes. There's no doubt, the female transition is a challenge both mentally and physically. As hormones plummet, most of us experience hot flashes, rollercoaster moods, sleep disturbances, headaches, and/or urinary issues. I've coped with some these issues myself.

Some self-help books for women say menopause should be a "time of acceptance." When it comes to improved self-care and understanding, I agree. But when the implication becomes it's time to kiss your shapely physique goodbye, I find that insulting! A fit body is something I intend to maintain for life.

Numerous research and anecdotal studies demonstrate that a woman's coping techniques with menopause determine the future of her physique. Most importantly, the stresses of this transition need to be managed or the person may cope by exercising less and overeating — and packing on weight.

With the headaches, sleep deprivation and rollercoaster moods I experienced in my late 40s and early-to-mid 50s, I felt like I needed my exercise more than ever! I depended on it to bring me back into balance. Unfortunately, many of my friends and clients enduring this very taxing transition are drinking more alcohol and rushing to the doctor for prescriptions to mask the discomforts they're experiencing.

Although in some cases, hormone replacement or other treatments may be necessary to mitigate severe symptoms, I think relying too heavily on medication to treat every issue is a big mistake. Why pop pills for anxiety and sleeplessness when you can eat healthier and try meditation or yoga so you can reestablish your chemical balance naturally?

Avoiding exercise is the last thing you want to do during this period of time when women are most susceptible to bone loss. If anything, menopause is a good time to step up your exercise program and do more strength training — for the sake of bone and mental health. Whether insurance pays for it or not, many physicians recommend that you get your first dexa scan during this time to ensure you're not at increased risk for osteoporosis. Medicating to mitigate bone loss is more effective when the condition is caught early.

Many of my clients were employed during their "thin years." After relocating to an upscale active adult community, many began to dine out daily and sometimes multiple times a day.

Most didn't want to think about how many calories lurked in each restaurant meal or plate of food served at a friend's house, so they stopped being careful and they stopped weighing themselves.

Many social events revolved around food and alcohol, so temptation was constantly present. They found it easier to just overeat and tell themselves it didn't matter than to plan ahead or maybe even decline invitations that would sabotage their healthy lifestyle efforts.

Some clients have such active social schedules they say there's no time to exercise. Only they can make the decision to restructure their priorities. **My observations of the behavior of dozens of clients indicate that the main causal factor for weight gain is an increase in food and drink intake and a decrease in activity levels.** I also know many clients, neighbors, and friends who haven't gained an ounce since menopause. They are the people who never miss a workout and could easily identify kale or beets in the grocery store!

Let's discuss how you can join the ranks of my model clients. As I've mentioned, menopause is a time of tremendous hormonal change. Diet can affect hormonal balance in a positive or negative way. Eating a diet high in white flour, sugar, and other preservative-laden foods creates imbalances in the hormone insulin and the hormones adrenaline and cortisol.

Many studies conclude that high levels of cortisol, a hormone released during stressful situations, leads to weight gain, particularly in the midsection. During situations perceived as stressful, your sympathetic nervous system reacts with a "fight or flight" response. Menopausal women often feel anxious and stressed and sometimes experience sleep disturbances.[5] I have experienced both of these troubling symptoms in recent years, but I work hard to mitigate them.

Swimming, yoga, and meditation help me to control stress and I use chamomile tea and Yoga Nidra to help with sleep. When traveling, I sometimes take melatonin 30 minutes before I want to sleep to help me adjust to time zone changes.

A chronic release of stress hormones, which can occur whenever a person becomes unable to regulate stress, is very likely to result in undesirable body changes. If you feel like your mind is always operating in high gear as if you need to flee from an attacking tiger, it's time to get a handle on your stress before your cortisol levels go haywire. Controlling anxiety (in the most natural manner possible) can go a long way toward reducing uncomfortable menopausal symptoms as well as balancing body chemistry.

Some women turn to foods high in fat and carbohydrate to control cortisol levels.[6] Resist the temptation and replace that emotional eating habit with a healthier form of stress reduction. Exercise, journal writing, and mindful activities such as Yoga, Qigong, meditation and Yoga Nidra can greatly improve your ability to cope with stress and improve sleep quality. In addition to my chamomile tea and Yoga Nidra rituals, I avoid screen time for at least an hour before bed and sometimes take a hot shower or bath or massage some diluted essential oil (peppermint is one of my favorites) into the back of my neck before turning in.

Aging women also gain weight due to loss of muscle mass. The more muscle in your body, the more calories burned, even when you sleep. Strength training is your body's best defense against age-related muscle loss. Numerous researchers have stated that resistance training benefits menopausal women by improving strength, body composition and bone density.[1]

When it comes to aerobic exercise during menopause, higher intensity isn't necessarily better. Research indicates that moderate physical activity is the best medicine for menopausal symptoms. Women who participated in moderate-intensity physical activity reported higher menopausal quality of life (MENQOL) and a lower total number of symptoms than women engaging in low- or high-intensity physical activity.[8] Inactive women reported the highest frequency of symptoms and the greatest discomfort. Walking, hiking, cycling, running, and swimming are all examples of aerobic exercise.

Aside from reduced physical activity and poor dietary habits, pinpointing other reasons why women gain weight during menopause is an area of ongoing scientific investigation. In a study by Brown and colleagues of more than 8,000 Australian women between ages 45 and 55, researchers found that menopause was an independent risk factor for weight gain. Over five years, study participants gained an average of slightly more than 1 lb (0.5 kg) per year. [4]

After adjusting for biological and behavioral variables, the researchers found that less exercise, quitting smoking, hysterectomy, and spending more time sitting were also independently associated with weight gain.[4] This is very significant! We're only talking about a pound over the course of a year, which is equivalent to 3,500 calories. If you replace empty calories with fruits and vegetables and increase your daily activity level, you could easily offset that weight gain (and even lose some weight in the process).

Burning more calories with physical activity can help in the maintenance of a healthy weight. A study by Lee and colleagues of 34,000 women showed that those who exercised at moderate intensity for 60 minutes daily (without diet modifications) experienced about one-half as much weight gain as their sedentary counterparts. [7]

Don't become another foregone conclusion when it comes to menopause and weight gain. Thousands of women maintain a healthy weight for their entire lifespan. You can, too, if you make a commitment to change and follow the principles outlined in this book.

REFERENCES

1 - Bemben, D.A., N.L. Fetters, M.G. Bemben, N. Navabi, and E.T. Koh. 2000. "Musculoskeletal responses to high- and low-intensity resistance training in early postmenopausal women." *Medicine & Science in Sports & Exercise, 32*(11): 1949-57.

2 - Bernstein M, and N. Munoz 2012. "Academy of Nutrition and Dietetics. Position of the Academy of Nutrition and Dietetics: food and nutrition for older adults: promoting health and wellness." *J Acad Nutr Diet.* 112(8):1255-1277.

3 - Blanck H.M., M.L. McCullough, A.V. Patel, C. Gillespie, E.E. Calle, V. Cokkinides, D.A. Galuska, L.K. Khan, and M.K. Serdula. 2007. "Sedentary behavior, recreational physical activity, and 7-year weight gain among postmenopausal US women." *Obesity*. 15(6):1578-1588.

4 - Brown W.J., L. Williams, J.H. Ford, K. Ball, and A.J. Dobson. 2005. "Identifying the energy gap: magnitude and determinants of 5-year weight gain in midage women." *Obes Res*. 13(8):1431-1441.

5 - Coutinho de Azevedo Guimarães, A., and F. Baptista. 2011. "Influence of habitual physical activity on the symptoms of climacterium/menopause and the quality of life of middle-aged women." *International Journal of Women's Health, 3:* 319-328.

6 - Dallman, M.F., N. Pecoraro, S.F. Akana, S.E. la Fleur, F. Gomez, H. Houshvar, M.E. Bell, S. Bhatnagar, K.D. Laugero, and S. Manalo. 2003. "Chronic stress and obesity: A new view of 'comfort food.'" *Proceedings of the National Academy of Sciences, 100* (20):1696–701.

7 - Lee I.M., L. Djoussé, H.D. Sesso, L. Wang, and J.E. Buring. 2010. "Physical activity and weight gain prevention." *JAMA*. 303(12):1173-1179.

8 - Luque, M. 2011. Physical activity and quality of life through the menopausal transition. Unpublished dissertation. Trident University International.

CHAPTER SIX

Diet Analysis: Quantity and Quality

Most of my incoming personal training clients said they wanted to lose weight. They also often said they didn't know why they weren't thinner. People 50 or more pounds overweight often said, "I don't eat very much." When I suggested they keep a food journal for two days and bring it in for a brief review, they tended to thank me for the offer and then never follow through. Among the slew of excuses I heard in response to my reminders were "I'm too busy," "My eating habits are good, I just need to exercise" and "I can't lose weight because of my metabolism."

I asked people about night eating or whether they ate unhealthy snacks or consumed calories mindlessly. "No, I never do that," they said. At that point, I had reached a roadblock I couldn't break through.

I was able to provide them with an exercise program and help them improve their fitness, balance, flexibility and overall health. But I could do little to help reshape the physiques of these individuals.

The ugly truth is that you will almost never lose weight through exercise unless you also analyze and adjust your diet. It is also crucial to accept accountability for the shape you have. A metabolic disorder is rarely to blame and in every case, metabolism can be increased with regular exercise and by adding more movement throughout the day. If you reject my suggestion of scrutinizing your current dietary habits, analyzing them, and transforming them to what can work for weight loss and maintenance, this book will not help much.

I understand why people are afraid to keep a journal and place what they're eating under the microscope for analysis. There's the denial factor. None of us want to admit our diets need serious resuscitation and that fingers can't honestly be pointed at metabolism or a thyroid disorder or any current medication.

We alone are responsible for the shape we're in. And it's scary to make major lifestyle changes. I know because I made one many years ago when I made a commitment to healthy eating and another recently when I decided to retire early and spend most of my time in Mexico.

It's scary to write down what you're eating when you think the trainer or dietician might give you a condescending smile and make you feel bad about yourself. I know because clients who succeeded told me their concerns! I always did my best to assure them I would look at this information without judgment, that I would be analyzing what they were eating out of an effort to help them become healthier.

With the right trainer, harsh judgment should never be an issue. Most of us simply want to help others live better quality and healthier lives and that's what's propelled us to work in this field.

As I shared in my personal story earlier, I have had many people make me feel worthless and ashamed over my weight. And not all trainers adopt my approach of supportive encouragement. Some tend to be more critical or to adopt more of a hardball approach. I don't believe physicians, trainers and counselors should make you feel bad about yourself. And most of them won't. If they do, I recommend you seek out professionals who are more empathetic or perhaps have faced weight issues once themselves.

I hope you don't find anything I write in this book intimidating. I do hope you find it encouraging. I'm basically saying if I can do it and if many of my clients can do it, so can you! I'm here to help you. But you can't fix what's broken until you actually know what's wrong. And that's what a food journal can do for you.

The amazing news is that you can feel better within days if you adopt healthier eating habits! A 2016 *American Journal of Public Health* article following more than 12,000 participants showed that increased fruit and vegetable consumption was predictive of increased happiness, life satisfaction, and well-being. The study concluded that "happiness" gains from healthy eating occur quickly and often many years before people experience enhanced physical health.[1]

If you're willing to keep reading, that's a good start. Remember, losing weight is all about energy balance. If you feed your body more than it burns in a day, the excess energy will be stored as fat and you will gradually gain weight. Any day you give the body less food than it uses for exercise, bodily functions and daily living tasks, your fat stores will serve as fuel and you will gradually lose weight.

Hopefully, after reading the *Fitter Than Ever* guidelines, you began keeping a food journal. If you are still telling yourself there's no way you want to do that, please bear with me because breaking through the fear and denial associated with this process and reconstructing your eating habits will literally change your life.

If I've convinced you to pursue the food journal, why not start today? Without "trying to be good" or intentionally eating less, please eat what you normally do and record it all for at least *two weeks*. When you don't record what you're eating, your mind might not process calories you eat in your car on the way to work or any nibbling that goes on while preparing dinner. That's why many people have the misperception that they "don't eat that much." Once you identify the foods you are eating and the quantities and then compute the calories, you can identify problem areas with your eating and start making changes.

Remember to write down the dough you lick from your fingers while baking cookies and the cookie crumbs you eat from the cookie tin so "they don't go to waste." Most of my clients that kept a food journal were shocked at how many calories slipped by their radar. Although it can be startling to see, many people found it encouraging as well. Some said they wished they'd done it much earlier.

It is frustrating to feel doomed to obesity by a metabolic disorder, yet not so difficult to accept change may be necessary if it won't leave you hungry or deprived. When what's recorded shows that you really are eating more than you thought, you realize that you could easily trim down some those "mindless" calories without even noticing. And this is fabulous news!

Once you record the initial two weeks of eating as recommended in Chapter One, pull out your red marker and write all over your food log. Where can you replace white with wheat? When can you choose to have a piece of fruit over a slice of cake? Can you start cooking with olive oil instead of vegetable oil for heart health? Can you replace that 200-calorie soda with water or green tea?

Figure out what you need to amend or decrease total caloric consumption to reach your TDEE (total daily energy requirement) - 500 (or TDEE - 750) and to enhance nutritional benefits. Then continue to record and follow the recommendations from Chapter One until it becomes second nature to eat a healthy, well-balanced diet with minimal "empty" calories.

LifeSum, SparkPeople, MyNetDiary, MyFitnessPal, LoseIt!, CarbManager, and ControlMyWeight are highly rated apps (for 2021) that you can install on your smart phone to make tracking your food easy. Many of them have extensive databases of food items and then you are able to add other foods as well. The foods in the databases include extensive nutritional information.

Determining quantities at first can be tricky. You may want to invest in a digital food scale. By using that and measuring cups for a while, you can eventually learn to eyeball quantities accurately, so you don't have to measure or weigh each time. Measure as much as possible in the beginning and then estimate once you feel you have a good concept of portions.

REFERENCES

1 - Mujcic, R. and A.J. Oswald. 2016. "Evolution of Well-Being and Happiness After Increases in Consumption of Fruit and Vegetables." *Am J Public Health.* 106(8): 1504-10.

CHAPTER SEVEN

Nutrition 101*

Although much of the content of this chapter may be familiar or repetitive to you, I have assembled it to enhance your ability to make healthy eating choices. You can find more nutritional information online at myplate.gov. The three major macronutrients our body needs to sustain life are carbohydrates, proteins and fats.

Carbohydrates

Do yourself a favor and forget the notion that carbohydrates are "bad." People develop a fear of them because consuming the wrong ones in large quantities can expand your waistline and harm your health. However, eating the right carbohydrates can mean the difference between a lousy day and a great one! And carbs can provide energy for your workouts.

Start to evaluate the carbohydrates you are consuming and aim for quality. The carbohydrates to avoid are cakes, pies, and other sugary desserts. Also avoid or minimize any foods that contain refined sugar or high fructose corn syrup.

Many foods people think of as healthy, such as whole grain breads and cereals can have a high sugar content. Learn to read labels and if you eat cereal in the morning, consider changing to oatmeal or making your own lightly-sweetened granola.

Many vegetables and fruits are high in carbohydrates and because they are also high in nutritional content and illness-preventative, they should make up the lion's share of your diet.

One gram of carbohydrates contains 4 calories. Carbohydrates serve as fuel for your body, especially your muscles and brain. Once carbohydrates are broken down and stored in the muscles and liver as glycogen, you will be able to use them as energy, which will enable you to work out for a sustained amount of time without fatigue.

Eliminating too many carbohydrates from your diet will leave you feeling mentally and physically exhausted. You may experience mood swings, fatigue, and even body-aches if you cut back on them too much. I did follow a KETO protocol for about two years, which strictly limits carbohydrates, to aid with a physical condition. It takes days or weeks to adjust to this way of eating and I recommend you only embark on this way of eating if you have a solid reason (treatment for seizures, migraine and other neurological diseases, appetite management). I used the Carb Manager App to track my carbohydrate consumption while I was following this protocol.

Carbohydrates are comprised of sugar molecules or saccharides. Monosaccharides and disaccharides are considered simple sugars because they are comprised of one or two sugar molecules. Glucose, fructose, and galactose are examples of simple sugars.[1,2] These simple carbohydrates are the ones that have given carbohydrates a bad rap.

Many people think these starchy foods are fattening. They aren't. But some, such as croissants, breakfast rolls, cakes, and muffins, offer few vitamins and minerals per calorie and may leave you craving another sugar high within the hour. Sedentary people tend to suffer more health problems (and weight gain) when they consume too many simple carbohydrates compared to very active individuals, whose bodies have adapted to rapidly transform available sugar into muscle fuel.

The old USDA food pyramid positioned breads, rice and other grains at the base, encouraging people to consume more carbohydrates than other foods. This may have contributed to many sedentary Americans gaining weight.

Since the 1980s, when the USDA first released this carb-based food pyramid, obesity and type 2 diabetes has more than doubled. [14] It simply isn't healthy to eat a diet rich in starchy carbohydrates if you're not doing any activity to burn them off.

Many simple carbohydrate-rich foods also contain added fat. Even if your slice of sourdough bread is relatively low in fat and calories, if you pour or spread on fats like margarine, oil, mayonnaise, cheese sauce or gravy, the calories multiply.

Foods high in sugar (as well as fat and salt) are often classified as hyperpalatable. These foods trigger addictive responses in the brain so that you crave more of them, whether you're hungry or not.[9] Over the course of months or years, you will lose a taste for real food, eating more of this food low in nutrients. These preservative-laced foods will leave you feeling like total crap (and with an expanded waistline).

Sugar molecules linked together into a long chain (oligosaccharides and polysaccharides) are called complex carbohydrates. The body has to work harder to break down complex chains of sugar molecules. These are the good guy carbohydrates you want to start eating more of instead of the nutrient-poor simple carbohydrates.

Cellulose or plant fiber is a complex carbohydrate. It gives your digestive system a workout in a good way – supporting its function while burning extra calories in the process. This fiber passes through the body without being absorbed, exercising the colon, improving motility and eliminating toxins and substances that can raise blood cholesterol levels. [1]

Complex carbohydrates give you a sense of fullness that lasts for hours, unlike a quick cookie or can of soda. Some complex carbohydrates, including oats and bananas, stimulate healthy bacteria in the gut.

Wheat, rice, oats, cornmeal, and barley are complex carbohydrates. Many fruits and vegetables include both simple and complex carbohydrates. Whole-grain foods contain the entire grain kernel: bran, germ and endosperm. Examples include oatmeal, bulgur, whole wheat flour, whole cornmeal and brown rice.[7]

White flour, white rice and pasta are examples of refined grains, which have been milled to remove the bran and germ. This processing gives grains a finer texture and improves their shelf life, but it also removes dietary fiber, iron, and many B vitamins. Often these refined grained are enriched or have these nutrients added back after processing. [7]

Choose your carbohydrates wisely and you'll feel full longer and experience fewer cravings.

Glycemic Index of Carbohydrates

Glycemic index (GI) is a numeric measure from 0 to 100 of how quickly blood glucose levels rise after eating a food. Foods like candy, white bread, and white rice have high glycemic indices because they are rapidly absorbed into the bloodstream. Whole grains or complex carbohydrates that take longer to digest have low glycemic indices (55 or less). [1]

Most junk food has high GI ratings. Some vitamin-rich foods are also on the high glycemic index list, including beta-carotene-packed carrots and cantaloupe. Am I telling you to give up cantaloupe and carrots? Not unless your physician advises you to do so! But be careful about eating too many foods with a high glycemic index because they can take a toll on your health.

Sodas, alcohol, cookies, crackers, biscuits, rolls, ice cream, and white bread can wreak havoc on healthy blood sugar levels. Try to keep them to a minimum. You're thinking you've got to be kidding. Okay, so maybe you don't have to completely eliminate these items, but if you are serious about losing weight and improving or maintaining your health, keeping blood sugar stable should be high on your priority list. Remember, in general, the less active you are, the more hazardous simple sugars are for your health!

The body releases insulin in response to sugar entering the bloodstream. If insulin levels rise to an excessive level, blood sugar will at first rise to a peak and then abruptly drop. Anytime this happens, you will generally feel tired, irritable and hungry. So before long, you are eating again and because of the generally lousy feeling, you may turn to comfort foods to give you another "pick me up."

Excess sugar that can't be used by the body and muscles is converted to triglycerides in the liver. In addition, this excess blood sugar causes bodily inflammation known as "glycemic stress." Spiking blood sugar levels that occur repeatedly over a period of too many years can lead to insulin resistance. The pancreas must release large amounts of insulin to combat excessive blood sugar levels caused by eating too many simple carbohydrates or too much food in general.

Eventually, the insulin receptors in the cells lose their ability to respond "normally" and blood sugar is no longer properly regulated. Excess blood sugar is stored as fat (not only around the belly and hips but in the arteries and heart) and eventually the person may develop Type 2 diabetes. You may also develop what Ray Strand, M.D. has coined Syndrome X or Metabolic Syndrome, a condition characterized by central obesity (excessive belly fat) and increased risk for Type 2 diabetes and heart disease. [6,9]

In addition to helping with weight loss and diabetes prevention, a diet that stabilizes blood sugar will give you more energy, improved cognitive ability, less hunger, fewer hot flashes and other menopausal symptoms, and better moods. Isn't it worth giving up some favorite "bad" foods, which you enjoy for only a minute, for feel-good benefits, which stay with you all day?

Some examples of high glycemic index items are:

Apple juice

White rice

Potatoes

Cake

Candy Bar

Distilled spirits

Jam

Pasta

Sugar

Syrup

Waffle

Bagel

Doughnut

Wine

Some examples of low glycemic index foods (with an index less than 55) are:

Apples

Rye bread

Cauliflower

Green Beans

Lentils

Cabbage

Mushrooms

Broccoli

Onions

Oats

Peaches

Grapes

Pasta (ranges from 50-55)

In general, fruits and vegetables, beans, less processed grains, low-fat dairy, and nuts tend to fall in the low GI category. For a more comprehensive list of foods and glycemic index, go to http://www.the-gi-diet.org/lowgifoods/

Protein

Protein is a constituent of muscle, bone, skin, hair and every other tissue in your body. When digested, protein is broken down into amino acids, which are used to replace and restore damaged tissues. One gram of protein contains 4 calories. If you don't eat enough protein when exercising, you may lose muscle mass. Recent studies following protein consumption of a population of people ages 52 to 75 years old found that higher protein consumption helped build muscle. The most favorable muscle building occurred for those consuming 1.2 to 1.5 grams of protein (per day) per pound of body weight. [4]

Yet, the average American consumes too much meat. If you find yourself eating meat at every meal, try replacing some meat proteins with plant proteins, which are equally rich in bodybuilding amino acids. Eating about 30 grams of protein during a meal maximizes protein synthesis (muscle building) rates.[10]

Try to select meat protein sources with less saturated fat. The best sources of protein from meat include fish and seafood (bass, cod, clams, haddock, halibut, lobster, salmon, shrimp, sardines, snapper, swordfish, tuna, trout), chicken breast, and turkey. Meats to be avoided include bacon, salami, pepperoni, hot dogs, and sausage. How the meat is prepared and cut also affects saturated fat content. Go for grilled, broiled or baked over fried and choose lean cuts of meat. Other good sources of protein include dairy, eggs, and tofu.

Animals raised on wild grasses (instead of heavily sprayed corn) and that have room to roam end up as leaner, healthier meat on your plate. "Ranch raised" meat products, though notably more expensive, are healthier for you in many ways not only because they contain less fat but also because they don't contain hormones or antibiotics.

Grass-fed meats are available and clearly marked at Trader Joe's, Whole Foods, and Sprouts. Do your body and the environment some good and choose these meat products over the poorer quality, less expensive ones.

Vegetarians can glean sufficient protein from a plant-based diet. At this time, I do not recommend consuming "plant-based" meat products, which contain more chemicals than anything else. Most contain few real plant products, are very high in sodium, and contain harmful additives such as food dyes (red #3, red #40 and caramel coloring), TBHQ, STPP, and methylcellulose.[18]

Every one of us can benefit from sinking our teeth into some of these plant-based foods, which are packed with nutrients and protein. [3]

Edamame (9 grams of protein per 1/2 cup, cooked)

Tempeh (16 grams per 3 ounce serving)

Tofu (8-15 grams per 3 ounce serving)

Lentils (8 g per 1/2 cup serving, cooked)

Quinoa (8 g per 1 cup serving, cooked)

Black beans (8 grams per 1/2 cup serving, cooked)

Lima beans (5 grams per 1/2 cup serving, cooked)

Peanuts (8 grams per ounce)

Red Potatoes (7 grams per large potato, cooked)

Refried Beans (6.5 grams per 1/2 cup serving)

Wild Rice (6.5 grams per cup serving)

Chickpeas (7 grams per 1/2 cup serving)

Almonds (6 grams per 1/4 cup serving)

Chia seeds (6 grams per 2 tablespoons)

Steel cut oatmeal (5 grams in 1/4 cup - dry)

Cashews (5 grams per 1/4 cup serving)

Pumpkin seeds (5 grams per 1/4 cup serving)

Sweet Potatoes (5 grams per 1 large potato, cooked)

Green Peas (4 grams per 1/2 cup serving, cooked)

Soybean Sprouts (4 grams per 1/2 cup serving, cooked)

Spinach (3 grams per 1/2 cup serving cooked)

Corn (2.5 grams per 1/2 cup serving)

Artichokes (2.5 grams per 1/2 cup, cooked)

Snow Peas (2.5 grams per 1/2 cup, cooked)

Avocado (2 grams per 1/2 avocado)

Broccoli (2 grams per 1/2 cup serving, cooked)

Brussels Sprouts (2 grams per 1/2 cup serving, cooked)

Asparagus (2 grams per 1/2 cup serving, cooked)

White mushrooms (2 grams per 1/2 cup serving, cooked)

Fat

Fat, composed of carbon atoms bonded together to form compounds known as fatty acids, supplies the body with 9 calories per gram of food consumed compared to 4 for protein and carbohydrates. Aim to eat about 35 percent of your total calories from fat and to consume primarily healthy (non-saturated) fats.

You may be thinking, wait? 35 percent? But I thought fat was bad for you! Fat has been slated as the enemy on the USDA food pyramid for years. Studies are increasingly showing that sugar and processed carbohydrates are your worst enemy and fat can actually be your friend. Fat offers many health benefits, if chosen wisely and in the proper quantities.

Consumption of fat with meals can provide you with a sustained sense of fullness. However, too much fat consumption can lead to weight gain. The wrong kind of fat in the diet can lead to heart disease. Some people who eat only moderate amounts of food are unable to lose weight because they add too much fat to meals in the form of calorie-dense condiments and sauces. Added fats in the form of trans fats are very harmful.

There are three different kinds of fats: monounsaturated, polyunsaturated, and saturated. Monounsaturated and polyunsaturated fats are liquids at room temperature. Monounsaturated fats occur in vegetable and nut oils such as olive, peanut, and canola as well as olives, cashews, almonds, and avocados.

Polyunsaturated fatty acids are most abundant in corn, soybean, safflower, cottonseed, fish, and sunflower oils.

Saturated fats, which are found in most animal products, can raise the LDL (bad cholesterol) levels, if consumed in excess.[1]

Unsaturated fats like vegetable oil can be transformed into a saturated fat through a process called hydrogenation. Hydrogenated fats are commonly referred to as trans fats on nutritional labels. These trans fats are solids at room temperature and consuming them can lead to plaque build-up in the blood vessels.

Trans fat or hydrogenated or partially hydrogenated fats should never be consumed. They are a major threat to heart health. [1,15]

Vegetable shortening and many salad dressings, vegetable oils (soybean, corn, canola), margarines, microwave popcorn packages, store-bought frozen pizzas, pies, cookies, and cakes, crackers, canned frosting, and non-dairy creamers contain artery-clogging trans fat. All are high in calories. Read the ingredient list even if the label says 0 grams of trans fat. If partially hydrogenated fat appears on the label, do not buy the food item! [16]

Many restaurants cook with vegetable oil laced with trans fat because its inexpensive. Aim to order foods that are grilled, not fried, or ask the server how your desired dish will be cooked and request that your food be specially prepared if necessary.

When you need a fat to flavor or cook food, I recommend olive oil as your go to. It is healthy and stays relatively stable at high temperatures (high smoke point). Butter, coconut oil, avocado oil, and hazelnut oil are also safe for cooking and can be used in moderation.

Fruits and Vegetables

A 2006 *Journal of the American Dietetic Association* reported that Americans eat much fewer than the recommended daily servings of fruits and vegetables. [5] A 2012 article in the *American Journal of Public Health* reiterated the inadequacy of fruit and vegetable consumption in the American diet.[12] These nutrient-dense, disease-preventing foods are vital for good health! Shunning them leads to approximately 2.6 million deaths per year.[6]

Avoiding fruits and vegetables is a very poor lifestyle choice. Multiple studies show abundant consumption of fruits and vegetables improves mood and sense of well-being as well as lowering the risk for many diseases and illnesses.

Fruits provide vitamins, carbohydrates, and fiber. They are low in calories and naturally sweet. Mangoes, papayas, melons and citrus fruits, like oranges and grapefruit, are high in vitamin C. Cantaloupe, apricots, peaches, and nectarines are good sources of vitamin A.

Whole fruits like apples and grapes contain more fiber than fruit juices. Dried fruits such as figs, prunes and raisins are good sources of fiber. Choose canned or frozen fruits packed in their own juice instead of syrup whenever fresh fruit isn't readily available.

Vegetables are an excellent source of vitamins, minerals and carbohydrates. In general, the more colorful the veggie, the more antioxidants you get in every bite. Antioxidants fight cellular damage from free radicals and can reduce the incidence of heart disease, cataracts, macular degeneration, and some cancers. [13] Organic vegetables picked when ripe are the richest in nutrients.

There are five different types of vegetables: dark green, orange, dry beans and peas, starchy vegetables, and other vegetables. Because vegetables differ in the vitamins and minerals they contain, it is important to eat a variety of them. Cabbages, plantains, peppers and leafy green vegetables are rich in vitamin C. Deep orange and dark green vegetables are high in vitamin A. The cruciferous leafy green vegetables broccoli, spinach, collards, cabbage, and kale contain calcium and iron and eating them may inhibit the growth of certain cancers.

Plant foods like lentils, black-eyed peas, chick peas and other dried beans and peas are inexpensive sources of protein. Unlike meats, beans are low in fat and high in fiber.

Nuts can tamp down hunger, are a great source of nutrients, contain polyphenol (which act as antioxidants), and reduce disease risk factors when consumed regularly.

Almonds are rich in Vitamin E and magnesium and support gut health. Hazelnuts are also Vitamin E- and magnesium-rich. Pistachios may reduce the rise of blood sugar after a meal. Walnuts may reduce inflammation that can lead to a host of chronic diseases. Cashews may reduce blood pressure and boost HDL (good) cholesterol levels. Macadamia nuts offer a host of heart-healthy benefits.

Nut butters such as peanut and almond butter are good sources of protein and iron; but they contain more saturated fats than nuts alone, so pay attention to serving sizes.

Some nut butters contain added oil and sugar, so read labels carefully. Your best bet is to buy all-natural nut butters. [17]

Meat, Poultry, Fish, and Eggs

The meat group nourishes your body with protein, iron, zinc, and the B-complex vitamins thiamin, riboflavin, niacin, B6 and B12. Meats are excellent sources of protein and contain all the essential amino acids your body needs for optimal health.

Some meat cuts and meat products are high in fat. Emphasize meat and poultry choices that are lean or low in fat. Grass-fed beef is available and clearly marked at Trader Joe's, Whole Foods, and Sprouts. Do your body and the environment good and choose these products over the poorer quality, less expensive ones.

To reduce fat, choose leaner cuts like chuck, bottom round or top round of beef, pork loin or lamb shank and eat poultry and fish more often. Always drain fat from meat before eating or adding additional ingredients. Contemporary studies continue to link consumption of red meat (particularly when grilled at high temperatures) to heart disease and cancer. It is recommended that you consume red meat infrequently.

Fish are high in Omega-3 fatty acids, which have been shown to fight depression, improve eye health, reduce heart disease risk, fight inflammation, and prevent cancer. Be sure to eat them at least once a week.

Avoid high-in-fat-and-sodium processed meats like hot dogs, sausage, pepperoni, bacon, ham and lunchmeats. If buying meat substitutes, read labels carefully to ensure they don't contain harmful ingredients before purchasing.

Eggs are an inexpensive source of protein. They're also rich in selenium, Vitamin D, B6, B6, zinc, iron, and copper.

Milk, Yogurt and Cheese

Dairy products are the best sources of the mineral calcium and also provide vitamin D, protein and phosphorus. Some milk products like ice cream, cheese, whole milk and foods derived from whole milk are high in saturated fat. Fat and calories can be minimized by choosing low-fat or non-fat versions of these products. Whole milk is much higher in Omega-3 fatty acids than lower fat milks and may be beneficial to include in your diet in small amounts once ideal weight is achieved.

*Always consult with your physician for appropriate guidelines on diet for your specific health needs. This book in no way substitutes for or constitutes medical advice.

REFERENCES

1 - Balch, P. 2010. *Prescription for Nutritional Healing Fifth Edition: A Practical A-to-Z Reference to Drug-Free Remedies Using Vitamins, Herbs, and Food Supplements.* New York: Avery (a member of Penguin Group).

2 - Carpi, A. 2003. "Carbohydrates." Vision Learning. 3(3). http://www.visionlearning.com/en/library/Biology/2/Carbohydrates/61

3 - Eckelkamp, S., and J. Smith. 2021. "20 High-Protein Vegetables to Add to Your Diet According to Dieticians." *Prevention online.* https://www.prevention.com/food-nutrition/healthy-eating/a20514733/high-protein-vegetables-and-plant-based-food/

4 - Fetters, A. 2015. "Older Adults: Double Your Protein for Better Health." *U.S. News and World Report online* (http://health.usnews.com/health-news/health-wellness/articles/2015/02/13/older-adults-double-your-protein-intake-for-better-health)

5 - Guenther, P.M., K.W. Dodd, J. Reedy, and S.M. Krebs-Smith. 2006. "Most Americans eat much less than recommended amounts of fruits and vegetables." *J Am Diet Assoc.* 106(6):1371-1379.

6 - Lock, K., J. Pomerleau, L. Causer, D.R. Altmann, and M. McKee. 2005. "The global burden of disease attributable to low consumption of fruit and vegetables: implications for the global strategy on diet." *Bull World Health Organ.* 83(2):100-108.

7 - MyPlate.gov (https://www.choosemyplate.gov/grains)

8 - Patterson, B.H., G. Block, W.F. Rosenberger, D. Pee, and L.L. Kahle. 1990. "Fruit and vegetables in the American diet: data from the NHANES II survey." *American Journal of Public Health.* 80(12): 1443-1449.

9 - Reaven G. 2000. *Syndrome X.* New York: Simon and Schuster.

10 - Peeke, P. 2012. "The Dopamine Made Me Do it." *IDEA Fitness Journal.* 9(9): 34-42.

11 - Symons, T. B., M. Sheffield-Moore, R.R. Wolfe, and D. Paddon-Jones. 2009. "A moderate serving of high-quality protein maximally stimulates skeletal muscle protein synthesis in young and elderly subjects." *Journal of the American Dietetic Association.* 109(9): 1582-1586.

12 - Whitehead, R.D., G. Ozakinci, I.D. Stephen, and D.I. Perrett. 2012. "Appealing to Vanity: Could Potential Appearance Improvement Motivate Fruit and Vegetable Consumption?" *American Journal of Public Health.* 102(2): 207-11.

13 - Willcox, J., S. Ash, and G. Catignani. 2004. "Antioxidants and Prevention of Chronic Disease." *Critical Reviews in Food Science and Nutrition.* 44(4): 275-295.

14 – Karlan-Mason, G., and R. Shi. 2020. "The Food Pyramid and How Money Influences USDA Dietary Guidelines." *GreenChoice.* https://www.greenchoicenow.com/v/food-pyramid-usda-dietary-

15 – Mozaffarian, D., A. Aro, and W.C. Willett. 2009. "Health effects of trans-fatty acids: experimental and observational evidence." *Eur J Clin Nutr.* 63(2): S5-21.

16 – Coyle, D. 2018. "7 Foods That Still Contain Transfats." *Healthline online.*
https://www.healthline.com/nutrition/trans-fat-foods

17 – Robertson, Ruairi (2018). "The Top 9 Nuts to Eat for Better Health." *Healthline online.*
http://www.healthline.com/nutrition/9-healthy-nuts

18 –Clean Food Facts Blog. "Are the new plant-based meats actually good for you?"
https://wellness.consumerfreedom.com/plant-based-meat/

CHAPTER EIGHT

Why Only Diet or Only Exercise (Usually) Won't Slim You Down

In a blog post entitled "Winning at Losing: Secrets of Long-Term Weight Loss," Dr. Len Kravitz shares studies by the National Weight Control Registry that consistently show that the people who lose weight and keep it off do the following on a consistent basis: 1) participate in high levels of physical activity, 2) Consume a low-calorie, low-fat diet and 3) weigh themselves frequently. A fourth common strategy most (78 percent) members reported is eating breakfast (typically cereal and fruit) every day.

Many people hired me for training and said they wanted to lose weight. Then they punctuated that statement by saying they didn't want to change what they ate. It was too inconvenient, or life was too short they would often say. Believe me, I understand this quandary. I've tried diet plans where it was almost impossible to have a social life and the recommended "food" tasted worse than wallpaper paste (yes, I actually sampled some as a toddler, but only once). I agree life's definitely too short to follow weight loss plans like those!

Unfortunately, weight loss is seldom achieved through exercise alone. Diet modifications are almost always requisite. The good news is that the *Fitter Than Ever* healthy lifestyle plan I've outlined for you isn't about deprivation and inconvenience. It's about making good food choices and teaching yourself to enjoy and prepare (without much trouble) food that's nourishing for your body and mind.

Here's the tricky part...Some of you will find that your taste buds have become so overstimulated from eating preservative-rich foods that you only crave more of the garbage that you most need to avoid. In these instances, you will have to train your taste buds to appreciate healthy food. This is achievable. It will, however, take some time and you will need to be patient. Nothing amazing happens overnight. Any worthwhile goal takes determination and persistence to attain.

Start by choosing one or two fruits or vegetables that you love and start to build on that. Then start to compile a list of healthy fruits and vegetables that you enjoy in your journal and look for recipes that include these foods.

Experiment with seasonings (I'm talking about real ones like turmeric, garlic, fennel, and oregano, not the ones loaded with mysterious substances).

Let's return to the discussion about why exercise alone rarely incites weight loss. The first issue is psychological. Many people engage in exercise they dislike and subconsciously think they "deserve" to eat more as a reward for the torture.

Exercise is a very inefficient way to "burn off" food. One piece of pie or glass of apple juice can easily counteract the calories burned during a workout. If a person feels especially entitled, he or she may actually gain weight after starting an exercise program. The truth of the matter is that this happens far too often. Finding enjoyable exercise will be one way you can remediate this counterproductive "food reward" behavior. Jump to my Slim for Life Secret #11 for more on this topic!

Secondly, the body has a way of settling into the status quo. Most people burn 200 to 400 calories during a workout. Your caloric expenditure will depend on your body weight, exercise modality, and intensity. You could exercise for weeks in this manner without losing an ounce. You may, however, gain some muscle mass (a very positive change).

Set point is to blame for the tendency for weight not to budge with "small" changes in lifestyle habits. Once we have maintained a weight for months or years, the body gets used to this and a shake-up is required to establish a new normal. The good news is that once you lose weight and maintain it for a few months, it won't be a battle anymore to keep it off.

A slimmer body will become your new set point and then as long as you don't derail too far from your new eating and activity program, your weight will remain stable. The key is to not make this "shake-up" you need to lose weight too extreme.

Restricting calories too extensively results in sudden weight loss that throws the body into a tailspin. In their review of *The Biggest Loser* contestants' results, Fothergill et al. (2016) explained that extreme exercise and diet slow the body's resting metabolic rate (number of calories burned daily), encouraging the body to regain lost weight.[2]

Most overly restrictive diets throw your metabolism out of whack. Basically, the body has no time to adapt to the sudden weight drop and so it fights to restore what it interprets as normal—your current weight—and to prevent what it interprets may be happening—you're starving and need to conserve calories.

Some exercise haters embark on diets without getting up from their chairs. I'm not an advocate of this method, primarily because if you don't exercise, it will be very difficult for you to eat enough food to obtain sufficient nutritional balance and still lose weight. You also are likely to feel deprived because you will have to limit your caloric intake much more than an active individual.

I, along with countless fitness professionals, physicians and health care professionals, believe exercise is essential for health. Research studies also show that most people who lose weight and keep it off do so through regular exercise and healthy eating. By exercising while you change your eating habits, you can eat more and still lose weight while doubling your chances of losing the weight and keeping it off for life!

Some people assume since they only burn a few hundred calories during a workout, it will make no difference if they stop. A few hundred calories might not make much difference in one day, but over the course of a year burning an extra 500 calories a day could translate to the difference between maintaining your weight and gaining a whopping 48 pounds!

A similar amount of weight gain could occur if you suddenly decide you will stop in for a latte loaded with sugar and cream on the way to work every morning or devour a bowl of ice cream nightly after dinner. Keep this in mind before you reach for caloric energy drinks after exercising. What you need to do post-exercise is restore your muscles, not load your body up with excessive calories and sugar.

You might find eating differently difficult at first, but if you stick with it long enough, you will find that the benefits motivate you to continue. Eating healthy means feeding yourself with nutrients the body and brain need to function optimally instead of unknown chemicals that throw your entire system into fight or flight mode. Nourishing your body properly can improve sleep quality, mood, energy level, mental concentration, and help you lose weight.

REFERENCES

1 - Kravitz, L. "Winning at Losing: Secrets of Long-Term Weight Loss." (Blog Post)
https://www.unm.edu/~lkravitz/Article%20folder/winning.html

2 - Fothergill, E., J. Guo, L. Howard, J.C. Kerns, N.D. Knuth, R. Brychta, K.Y. Chen, M.C., Skarulis, M. Walter, P.J. Walter, and K.D. Hall. 2016. "Persistent metabolic adaptation 6 years after 'The Biggest Loser' competition." *Obesity*. 24(8): 1612-1619.
http://onlinelibrary.wiley.com/doi/10.1002/oby.21538/full

CHAPTER NINE

The Best Exercise: Cardiovascular and Strength Training Workouts for Weight Loss and Maintenance

The American College of Sports Medicine (ACSM) issues annual guidelines for exercise. The current (as of 2021) recommendations for healthy adults 18 to 65 are 5 or more days per week of a minimum of 30 minutes of moderate intensity exercise or 3 days or more days per week of high intensity aerobic exercise (minimum of 20 minutes). This translates to a minimum of 150 minutes of moderate intensity exercise or at least 60 minutes of high intensity exercise.

It is also recommended that adults perform exercises that maintain or improve muscular strength and endurance at least two times per week.[4,8]

It has been my experience that women over 40 achieve the best weight maintenance/weight loss results with 300 or more minutes of moderate intensity aerobic exercise each week. I know this sounds like a lot, but I'll show you ways to make this manageable even if you have limitations or an insane work schedule.

Three hundred minutes translates to 50 minutes, 6 days a week. ACSM also recommends training each muscle group two to three times per week, performing two sets of 8 to 12 repetitions to increase muscle strength and power. Regular strength training will reduce age-related muscle and bone loss.

I am unusual in that I exercise more than 600 hours a week. Here's a breakdown of my typical exercise week. I swim in the sea or pool 6 days a week for 45 minutes to an hour (moderate to intense 270 – 360 minutes), walk our Chow Chow for 60 minutes daily (low intensity 30 in the morning and 30 in the evening for a total of 420 minutes weekly) and teach yoga three times a week (180 minutes, which is my strength training since I use resistance bands in one class and body weight strengthening in the other two classes).

My weeks burst with activity. And I enjoy it! And the really good news... *My activity level enables me to eat whatever I want without gaining any weight.*

People often ask me what the best exercise is for weight loss. The simple answer is cardiovascular or aerobic exercise.

A more complex answer involves hunger and the number of calories burned during the exercise session. Someone who walks at a pace of one mile an hour for 60 minutes will obviously burn far fewer calories than someone who spends that hour running or exercising on an elliptical at a clipping pace.

I have personally found running to be the best exercise for weight loss. Any time I've wanted to drop a couple of pounds (after an indulgent vacation, for example), I've been able to do it by running more for a couple weeks. Jason Karp, the owner of Run-Fit, LLC and author of *Run Your Fat Off*, has helped hundreds of people lose weight through running. He has also authored numerous excellent resources on running, including my personal favorite, *Running for Women* (coauthored by Carolyn Smith).

"Running is so effective for weight loss because it demands a great need for energy," said Karp. "Only cross-country skiing supersedes running in its energy requirements. Running uses many muscles. The more muscles you use, the more calories you burn. It is accessible to everyone in the world."

Walking is another one of my weight loss favorites. I walked daily to keep from gaining excessive weight during both of my pregnancies because impact exercise caused back pain. If you want to up the ante on your walking routine, using more upper body and core muscles and reducing the stress on knees, hips and ankles, try Nordic Walking. With the support of Nordic walking poles (similar to ski poles) or similar equipment, you'll find it easier to go longer distances with less discomfort. You'll use more muscles, distribute weight more evenly, and find it easier to walk long distances without slouching into poor posture.

High Intensity Interval Training (HIIT) is a great way to burn beaucoup calories. Not only do you burn mega-calories while exercising, your caloric burn continues for hours afterward (see my Slim for Life Secret about excess post-exercise oxygen consumption or EPOC).

Swimming and water exercise, although amazing for heart health, relaxation and muscle tone, tend to be poor choices for weight loss. For one, water exercise tends to stimulate appetite. People also often don't work at a high enough intensity in the water to burn a significant number of calories. Floating on a noodle barely moving your arms and legs for an hour just doesn't cut it!

There are some exceptions to this rule. Very skilled swimmers burn almost as many calories as runners. I happen to be one of them! I also love the water. For people like us, it makes sense to swim often for exercise. Others, because of physical limitations, are restricted to water exercise. In these instances, dietary adjustments (keto or intermittent fasting) may be required to mitigate post-workout hunger. All of us are better off doing water exercise and/or swimming than parking ourselves in front of the TV. Use common sense when deciding what exercise is best for you.

Continuous exercise that elevates heart rate is good for your health and burns calories and fat. The advantage of adding strength training to your weekly workouts is that it builds muscle and strength and prevents rapid loss of muscle tissue than tends to occur with aging (sarcopenia). Strength training also is good for bone health.

Many women fear strength training, imagining that it will make them look masculine or unattractive. Because of this fear, they may try to do "shaping" workouts with useless one- or two-pound weights. These workouts won't increase your muscle mass or help you lose weight. Women don't build muscle the way men do because our hormones are different.

Ditch this fear of bulking up and pick up some real weights. Muscle burns more calories than fat, so it is your friend, not your enemy. If you've seen women who look masculine in the weight room, they are likely on steroids or are doing hypertrophy workouts, which are specifically designed to bulk up muscles.

Aim to work your major muscle groups: (quadriceps or the muscles in the front of thighs), hamstrings (back of thighs), glutes, deltoids (shoulders), pectorals (chest), back (latissimus dorsi and trapezius), biceps and triceps as outlined in Chapter One. Make sure you work the muscles hard to fatigue each time or the workout won't be effective. Increase weight gradually over the course of your training, so you continue to get stronger. Hiring a personal trainer can help you adhere to a program and stay safe.

REFERENCES

1 - Comana, F. 2012. "The Energy Balance Equation." *IDEA Fitness Journal*. 9(3).

2 - Douillard, J. 2001. *Body, Mind and Sport: The Mind-Body Guide to Lifelong Fitness and Your Personal Best*. New York: Three Rivers Press.

3 - Grattan, B.J., Jr., and J. Connolly-Schoonen. 2012. "Addressing weight loss recidivism: a clinical focus on metabolic rate and the psychological aspects of obesity." *ISRN Obesity*. https://www.ncbi.nlm.nih.gov/pmc/articles/PMC3914266/

4 – American College of Sports Medicine. 2021. "Physical Activity Guidelines." https://www.acsm.org/read-research/trending-topics-resource-pages/physical-activity-guidelines

5 - Manini, T.M. 2010. "Energy expenditure and aging." *Ageing Research Reviews.* 9(1): 1-11.

6 - Matthews, M. Muscle for Life website. https://www.muscleforlife.com/tdee-calculator/

7 - McMurray, R.G., J. Soares, C.J. Casperson, and T. McCurdy. 2014. "Examining variations of resting metabolic rate of adults: a public health perspective." *Medicine and Sciences in Sports and Exercise.* 46 (7): 1352-1358.

8 – Jakicic, J. 2019. "Physical Activity: A Key Lifestyle Behavior for Prevention of Weight Gain and Obesity." ACSM web site. https://www.acsm.org/all-blog-posts/acsm-blog/acsm-blog/2019/07/22/physical-activity-lifestyle-prevention-weight-gain-obesity

9 – Karp, J. and C. Smith. 2011. *Running for Women.* Champaign, IL: Human Kinetics.

10 – Karp, J. 2017. *Run Your Fat Off: Running Smarter for a Leaner and Fitter You.* Reader's Digest.

CHAPTER TEN

What If I Have Limitations?

Once age 50 strikes, most of us have physical limitations or at least have to be cautious doing certain activities. It's possible to work within your physical limits and still be very active. I see people doing that very thing every day of the week. At age 58, I have to be cautious with my right shoulder since I injured (and rehabilitated) a rotator cuff muscle in 2008. Far too often other parts of my body tell me I need to be more mindful. And I always listen!

Cardiovascular conditioning and strength training are your foundation for elevating heart rate, burning fat and calories and maintaining and/or building muscle mass. Some of you may be former athletes, while others of you may have never exercised. The table at the end of this chapter outlines some medical issues and the type of exercise most likely to be appropriate for you.

Please work with your body instead of fighting it. If your shoulder hurts, abort the swim workout and take a walk instead. If your knee is bothering you, consider a non-impact water workout. Most of the time, even when you're experiencing pain or have an active injury, you will be able to do some kind of activity that allows the trouble area to rest.

It is important to learn to recognize the difference between a muscle strain and delayed onset of muscle soreness (DOMS). DOMS, although uncomfortable, is not a serious condition and does not require any special treatment. It tends to peak 24 to 48 hours after activity and is characterized by discomfort in muscles that in some cases can last for several days.

An acute muscle strain tends to be felt during or immediately after activity and may be accompanied by swelling and skin discoloration.

Bursitis and tendonitis are other conditions of irritation and inflammation that can be experienced by overtraining athletes or new exercisers that push themselves too hard before they have achieved adequate conditioning.[1] In any of these instances, resting the painful area is warranted. Ice may help reduce muscular or joint inflammation and discomfort.

People who continue to force tired or strained tissues to work will often experience chronic strain as the injury progresses from minor to something more serious that may require medical intervention. For obvious reasons, halting the painful conditions in its early stages is a much more prudent choice!

The stationary recumbent bicycle is usually a good choice for people with back, knee and hip issues. Be sure to adjust the seat so that your knees never lock (they should be just slightly bent in the most extended part of the pedaling cycle).

Warm-water exercise (better with supportive footwear), suspended water running with an Aquajogger or similar vest, and swimming are the easiest on the body and are ideal modalities for people suffering from arthritis, fibromyalgia, or other painful joint and muscle conditions.

If you enjoy walking, hiking, running, and/or dance classes, be sure to buy supportive, quality footwear and replace it on a regular basis. Quality running stores will offer you a foot analysis, measuring foot length and width, arch height, and revealing whether you pronate or supinate. This will help you to buy a shoe right for your foot size and shape and running gait.

The analysis I received at Fleet Feet in northwest Tucson determined that I pronate slightly and had one foot slightly larger with a higher arch height. Adding a special insert to my Brooks running shoes balances my gait, reducing stress on my knees and ankles.

Impact exercise breaks down the cushioning in the shoes over time. My usual rule of thumb is to replace shoes every six months since I use them almost daily. Runners can use mileage as a rule of thumb for replacement (500 to 550 miles). My joints usually tell me when it's time to buy a new pair. If I take a run or a long walk and my knees, ankles or hips hurt afterward, that tells me the worn-out cushioning is no longer doing me much good.

Although I've included some guidelines for exercise, I highly recommend that you consult with your physician to discuss what is appropriate if you have serious medical issues. These guidelines are for reference only and are not meant to replace medical advice. Follow your physician's recommendations for activities and consult with your surgeon about any restrictions in activity post-surgery and timelines for returning to activity.

Hiring a personal trainer enables you to embark on a strength-training program that makes sense for your fitness level and medical conditions. This individual will review documents provided by your doctor and/or physical therapist and your health history before conducting a baseline assessment to determine your current level of fitness. The most highly qualified trainers have certifications from ACE (American Council of Exercise), AFAA (Athletics and Fitness Association of America), ISSA (International Sports Science Association), ACSM (American College of Sports Medicine), NSCA (National Strength and Conditioning Association), or NASM (National Academy of Sports Medicine).

During your initial meeting with your trainer, be prepared to share comprehensive information about your health including surgeries, orthopedic problems, medications, and current and past illnesses. You can take a list of medications with you to be attached to the form if there are too many to remember. Be sure to write down every single detail. If you fail to reveal something important, your trainer may inadvertently have you perform an exercise that could cause you harm.

I can't tell you how many times a client has filled out health history forms only to burst out mid-workout with, "Oh I almost forgot to tell you..." This tends to cause fitness professionals, including me, to break out in hives and have heart palpitations! One woman told me she'd had gall bladder surgery earlier that week after filling out her form (with no mention of the surgery) when we were headed to the weight room to begin training!

If your trainer asks (even after you've filled out the form), "Have you had recent surgery," or "Have you had a bone density test done recently," don't be offended. He or she, like me, probably just wants to make 100 percent sure for the sake of your safety that no vital health information was left uncovered.

Once you and your trainer have established safe guidelines for activity, you'll be given a cardiovascular and strength program to follow each week. The trainer will explain what to do and for how long and help you learn how to execute all strength training exercises properly. By doing the exercises in proper form, you are less likely to become injured. Your trainer will also function as a "support" person, helping you set goals, and offering encouragement and ways for you to measure your progress.

Establishing a comfortable relationship with your trainer will enable you to learn and readily improve. It's better not to become too chummy, though. Focus on each exercise session and avoid distracting conversations.

It can be tempting to release emotional baggage or initiate mindless chitchat during sessions. This will impair your results. When I was confronted with this, I didn't want to hurt feelings and often struggled to find tactful and compassionate ways to redirect clients back to the workout (because people were often talking about major concerns with health, loss, and personal relationships). There were occasions, of course, where the individual's need to talk took precedence and I honored that. After some light conversation, it is best to keep talk focused on the task at hand — asking whether your form looks good or possibly asking fitness or nutritional questions that you want answered.

Don't be offended if the trainer interrupts mid-sentence and asks you to focus. This is a good sign! Don't assume this trainer is insensitive and has no heart. In reality, it means the opposite. The responsible trainer, hired to help you improve your health and fitness, has simply recognized that the conversation is impairing his or her ability to teach you to do the exercises properly and realizes that the only way to effectively turn the situation around is to demand your full attention.

Much of your training will have to be done independently, especially the aerobic/cardiovascular training. Make sure you do what is asked of you. If your trainer tells you to do a 30-minute walk each day, do it. If your trainer gives you a stretch worksheet to follow daily, do it. If you do not adhere to the trainer's recommendations, you will not obtain the desired results. This reflects poorly on you and your personal trainer. Often trainers will not continue to work with clients who consistently cancel sessions or make excuses rather than doing what they are instructed to do.

Working with a personal trainer can be a very positive experience if you stay focused on your goals and why you are meeting the trainer in the first place. You will learn to exercise safely and have a person to encourage you and update you on the latest research in the health and fitness industry.

Table 4. Basic Safety Guidelines for Special Populations*

Condition	Recommended Activities	Activities to Avoid	Intensity
Cardiovascular Risk	Low intensity swimming, walking or stationary cycling	Running, cycling, high-intensity exercise without doctor's clearance	40 to 60 percent of maximum heart rate unless otherwise indicated by physician
Osteoporosis	Brisk walking, jogging, low impact aerobics, stair climbing	Non-impact, non-bone-building activities like swimming & cycling (as primary exercise). Avoid high impact activities, twisting, unsupported forward flexion, use of Smith machine or weighted vest without doctor's approval.	High-intensity preferable to strengthen bone tissue.
Fibromyalgia	Low impact activities such as swimming, walking, and cycling	High impact activities such as running and high impact aerobics	Low to moderate to avoid fatigue and muscle aches
Arthritis	Swimming and water exercise in warm water	High impact activities	Low to moderate to avoid joint discomfort
Asthma	Any enjoyable exercise. Do adequate warm-up and cool down. Wear face covering in cold conditions.	Outdoor activities when allergens high or air quality poor; poorly ventilated indoor facilities (swimming outdoors better since chlorine fumes don't accumulate)	Follow doctor's orders. Have inhaler available during workouts.
Diabetes	Low to moderate-intensity walking, swimming, or stationary cycling	Wear shoes during exercise activities.	Low to moderate: check blood sugar before and after exercise, drink plenty of fluids and stop if you feel dizzy

*Always consult with a physician before starting a new program.

REFERENCES

1 - Crews, L. 2006. "Injury Prevention: Group Strength." *IDEA Fitness Journal*. 3(10).

CHAPTER ELEVEN

Keto Diet and Time Restricted Eating (TRE)

In recent years, keto diets (where 70 to 80 percent of calories come from fat and carbohydrates are reduced most often to 20 to 50 grams per day) have become popular to lose weight. I pursued this way of eating for three years and can share some pros and cons based on personal experience. I'll also share what the research says.

I knew my diet needed to change. Several years ago, I began experiencing frequent indigestion, post-meal lethargy, and dizziness after drinking sports drinks or using gels for swimming competition. I was also constantly hungry, needing snacks almost every two hours. I wanted to be able to race without needing nutrition so often and without using gels and drinks that were full of chemicals. I wanted to travel without having to pack a bunch of food.

I found some online keto groups and they discussed how your body can be trained to burn body fat as energy instead of always relying on sugar, which enables you to go longer without food. That possibility excited me. Athletes said this versatility kept them from "bonking" during workouts or races. This also intrigued me since I have often had difficulty figuring out nutrition for all-day swimming competitions when racing every hour or so. Weight losers said they never suffered from uncomfortable hunger anymore. People suffering from migraines said it reduced their pain episodes. Done, sold. I decided to give it a try.

I started by downloading the Carb Manager app on my smartphone. This made it easy for me to figure out the fat, protein and carbohydrate content of different foods. After a few weeks, I had established a comfortable "norm" for eating.

Fortunately, I never suffered from the "Keto Flu." Some people new to this way of eating experience severe fatigue and body aches as a result of the dietary changes. Maybe I didn't experience this because I already had been largely avoiding sugar for many years and didn't have as extreme of an adjustment as some people may experience. I'm really not sure.

I initially suffered from constipation as my body adjusted to using vegetables and oils, rather than grains to facilitate smooth digestion. This lasted for about a month. I did find that if I was experiencing constipation that a tablespoon of olive oil would resolve the problem within an hour or so.

Eliminating grains turned out to be a lifesaver. Now I rarely experience what I often did before — diarrhea, bloating, and cramping. What a relief that has been.

During the time I was eating keto, and since I transitioned to a low-carbohydrate, sugar- and gluten-free diet (about five months ago), I usually exercise in the morning before eating and often after fasting for 12 or more hours. When I first started eating keto, I felt tired during workouts, especially when running when my legs felt leaden.

After a month or two, I became accustomed to training in ketosis and workouts became much more comfortable. Now I prefer fasting exercise it because I avoid the digestive upset I sometimes experienced when training within an hour or two after eating.

Within two weeks of starting keto, I was able to cut out snacks and soon noticed that I was rarely hungry even at mealtime. I am happy to say I haven't had a snack between meals in more than three years or even wanted one!

I shifted my breakfast time gradually until I was able to fast a minimum of 12 hours nightly and now, I most often fast daily for 15 or 16 hours. It became easy to wait for breakfast until 9, 10 or even 11 without uncomfortable hunger.

That's my story. Let's now look at what research says about ketogenic eating. In the 1920s, the high fat, low-carbohydrate diet was introduced as an effective treatment for children with epilepsy who had not responded to prescribed medications. More recently, it has been prescribed for diabetes, cancer, polycystic ovary syndrome, and Alzheimer's. This way of eating is now one of the most frequently followed diets for weight loss.[1]

On keto, dieters consume the lion's share of their calories from fat. Most carbohydrates, including all grains and starchy vegetables, are eliminated. Hello, ribeye steak, heavy whipping cream, and butter! After most carbohydrate-rich foods are removed, the body eventually runs out of glucose to use for energy and begins to rely on body fat as fuel.

When ketones are present in measurable quantities in the blood, this is known as ketosis. In the absence of glucose, ketones acetoacetate and B-hydroxybutyrate (BHB) provide energy for your heart, skeletal muscles, and brain. Ketones produce less inflammatory products as they are metabolized, and they reduce neuronal cellular damage. [6,7]

Many people report improved mental clarity and mood while in ketosis.

Anyone who goes for long periods of time without food will start to experience this shift to fat burning or state of ketosis. But most people eat so often, they rarely experience this.

Usually, the body will produce enough insulin on its own to keep the ketone levels from rising too high. The amount of ketone bodies that accumulate in the body depends on diet, how long the individual has gone without food and factors such as body fat percentage and resting metabolic rate. [1]

If your physician or nutritionist gives you the green light to try keto eating, please don't rush out and buy a bunch of "Keto" processed food items or start making high fat dessert recipes too often. This approach is a big mistake. Relying on sugar substitutes and eating processed food is unlikely to lead to weight loss and definitely won't improve your health. Your taste buds will continue to crave processed food and sweets.

Your best bet is to rely on real foods—meat, fish, nuts, whole fat dairy, legumes, fruits and vegetables for your foods and use natural seasonings to add flavor to foods. Soon you be satisfied eating real food and you will also start to notice the myriad benefits of eating a natural diet. Once you adapt to "real food" eating habits, it will be much easier to keep the weight you lose off without ever gaining it back.

For ideas on recipes, you can look online or purchase Keto cookbooks. One that I use often is *KETO Intermittent Fasting: 100 High-Fat Low-Carb Recipes and Fasting Guidelines to Supercharge Your Health.*

You can purchase monitoring kits such as the Keto Mojo to test your ketone and blood sugar levels. After a finger prick, a drop of blood on a strip gives you a reading on the monitor, so you can ensure your levels are within safe limits.

I used to test my blood sugar and ketones upon awakening, before meals, and then an hour or two after each meal. Once I adjusted to this way of eating, testing no longer was necessary. Consult with your physician about this process.

Research has shown following a keto protocol can result in weight loss as well as improved insulin resistance, decreased blood pressure, cholesterol, and triglycerides. [2, 3]

On the downside, following the diet is difficult, especially in social situations. I will confess, we got fewer invitations to dinner once friends and family learned about my way of eating.

Some people experience headaches, mood swings, fatigue and irritability on keto, although these symptoms often improve as a person's body adjusts to life with fewer carbohydrates. There is also an increased risk for osteoporosis and kidney stones.

In general, the keto diet is not recommended for people with complex health issues and is best done for a period of time and not indefinitely. Consult with your physician or a registered dietician before trying the keto diet. The nutritional specialist can ensure your choice of foods is well-balanced.

Boosting nutrition with a healthy array of vegetables, legumes and nuts can help to ensure a healthy balance of vitamins and minerals. Supplements may be recommended to ensure all necessary nutrients are covered. [1]

Many people who are unable to follow the keto diet can use time restricted eating (TRE) or fasting as tools to curb hunger and to gain some of the neuroprotective benefits of being in ketosis. Time restricted eating involves eating only during a window of 6 to 10 hours without restriction to caloric quantity or quality.

For more than a year, I did TRE while eating Keto. Now that I have shifted to no grains, no sugar, I continue to practice TRE.

A writer friend of mine reported losing 9 pounds in less than two months by narrowing her eating window alone!

Early research indicates TRE can lead to reduced body weight, improved glucose tolerance and metabolic flexibility, reduced atherogenic lipids and blood pressure, improved gut health and improved cardiovascular health. More research is needed to establish how this way of eating might benefit different populations. [4]

Other recent studies indicate that intermittent fasting increases cellular autophagy — or removal or "cleansing" of damaged cells in your body, which contribute to aging and neurological disease.[6,7]

A study of Muslims fasting during the Ramadan holiday indicated that fasting — particularly during daylight hours — may prevent osteoporosis by decreasing the Dipeptidyl peptidase (DPP-4) gene and activating the DPP-4 inhibitors.[8]

If you receive a green light to try TRE, you might gradually narrow your eating window to see how you adapt and then increase your period of fasting over time.

REFERENCES

1 – Diet Review: Ketogenic Diet for Weight Loss. Harvard School of Public Health.
https://www.hsph.harvard.edu/nutritionsource/healthy-weight/diet-reviews/ketogenic-diet/

2 – Paoli, A. 2014. "Ketogenic diet for obesity: friend or foe?" *Int J Environ Res Public Health*. 11(2):2092-2107.

3 – Schwingshackl, L., and G. Hoffman. 2013. "Comparison of effects of long-term low-fat vs. high fat diets on blood-

lipid levels in overweight or obese patients: a systematic review and meta-analysis." *J Acad Nutr Diet.* 113(12):1640-1661.

4 – Regmi, P., and L. Heilbronn. 2020. "Time Restricted Eating: Benefits, Mechanisms, and Challenges in Translation." *iScience.* 23(6): 101161.

5 – Stanton, B., and M. Anderson. 2020. *KETO Intermittent Fasting: 100 High-Fat Low-Carb Recipes and Fasting Guidelines to Supercharge Your Health.* Emeryville, CA: Rockridge Press.

6 – Jarreau, P. 2021. "The Five Stages of Intermittent Fasting." https://lifeapps.io/fasting/the-5-stages-of-intermittent-fasting/

7 – Alirezaei, M.; C. Kemball, C. Flynn, M. Wood, L. Whitton, and W. Kiosses. 2010. "Short-term fasting induces profound neuronal autophagy." *Autophagy.* 6(6): 702-710.

8- Kormi, S., S. Ardehkhani, and M. Kerachian. 2017. "The Effect of Islamic Fasting in Ramadan on Osteoporosis." *Journal of Fasting and Health.* 5(2):74-77.

CHAPTER TWELVE
Meditation and Yoga

In 2016, I flew to Big Corn Island, Nicaragua for a three-week yoga teacher training course. In recent years, I had recognized imbalance in my life. I was too focused on acquiring material possessions and had allowed my participation in Masters swimming to become too obsessive.

Every plan I made revolved around training and planning travel to national competitions. Always wanting one more thing I didn't have—a faster swim time, a newer car, another exotic vacation, a higher paying job, etc.—I found myself frequently ill, anxious, and depressed. I almost never experienced contentment in the moment. I was too busy looking ahead.

I wasn't spending enough quality time with family and friends. I found little joy in the pool. I knew that something had to change.

Yoga teacher trainings are most often done one of two ways—over the course of a series of weekends in the city where you live or as an immersion class. You can take an immersion class in almost any country you want to go.

Transitioning back and forth from real life to a series of weekend courses—exhausted after a long work week—seemed like it would be a chore, rather than a mindful journey. That wasn't what I wanted.

I chose to go away for the teacher training to immerse myself in the yogic lifestyle. I also selected a locale where I could swim every morning. I wanted to continue with daily exercise and thought sea swimming might revitalize my love for the water.

The teacher training experience turned out to be truly transformative. I swam through crystal clear water out to a reef every morning, rolling over on my back sometimes to watch the sun rise and puffy clouds turn colors. I felt so alive swimming—not in a chlorinated, man-made pool—but in open ocean, feeling the salt water embrace my skin and seeing so many colorful fish and other creatures too—a nurse shark, a group of spotted eagle rays.

It didn't matter what pace I swam. I wasn't trying to keep up with another person or race a time on the clock, I immersed myself in the sheer pleasure of moving through water. This love I had for open water swimming would inspire us to do a swim tour to the Ionian Islands in Greece and would lead me to swim almost daily once we bought our seaside condo on the Sea of Cortez.

My small, dark and dingy accommodations no longer bothered me by the third day. I felt so thrilled and grateful to be on this beautiful, remote island where I could connect with nature that my previous "need" to have a luxurious room now seemed silly.

Our two-hour morning Ashtanga practice was the part of the teacher training I enjoyed the most. No talking, no music, only the whisper of wind through leaves, birds singing and the occasional sound of a mango crashing down onto a bed of leaves in the underbrush.

I felt so peaceful and relaxed. And over the course of these weeks where I was away from my husband and my life in the States, spending hours each day in peaceful reflection, I started to really connect with myself. To understand. What I truly valued. What mattered to me. What I needed to thrive.

By the end of the teacher training, I realized I no longer wanted to live the typical American lifestyle. I craved simplicity, calm, spending quality time with family and friends. So often during the yoga teacher training, I'd flashed back to the two years I'd lived in Arequipa, Peru in the 1990s. I'd been happier and healthier there than ever before.

Life was slower-paced. I connected on a deep level with two Peruvians and several American friends I met while there. There were beautiful mountains and valleys and beaches to explore on foot and by mountain bike.

I wanted to have all that back again, to savor life in a slower-paced country. And after swimming in this sea for three weeks, I longed to be near the ocean. I felt so calm and serene around the water. Within a year, that dream began to take shape. We bought our condo in San Carlos, Mexico in August of 2017. We left behind the fancy house and the people rushing around worrying and struggling to get ahead and started living a slower-paced life.

My journey wasn't one of weight loss, but it was a journey to better self-understanding and finding a lifestyle that works better for my physical and mental well-being. People often fail to lose weight because they don't really understand themselves or what they need to do to motivate themselves toward change.

People who have been overweight for a long time sometimes have poor self-esteem, tend to stress eat, and have an uncomfortable relationship with food. All of these can be explored and often overcome through mindful practices. If this sounds impractical, read some of these research studies that have shown how yoga has transformed so many lives.

Most yoga practices burn fewer calories than cardiovascular exercise, so many people on weight loss journeys shy away from yoga classes. Yoga can provide low-impact cardiovascular exercise for clients who have suffered stress injuries from high-impact activities. It can also be used as "cross training" with other activities. Ashtanga and Vinyasa yoga classes involve many standing poses and flowing movements, which bring heat into the body, elevate heart rate, limber joints, and burn calories (about 460 per hour). Sun Salutations, a part of both of these practices, are particularly beneficial for burning calories and elevating heart rate.

You don't necessarily have to do a vigorous yoga practice to benefit, though. It is actually the mental and emotional shifts that often occur with regular practice that have been linked to weight loss.

In one study on yoga and obesity, 90 percent of the male and female subjects reported improved eating habits as a result of practicing yoga. Participants reported an increase in mindful eating, improvements in food choices, and decreased emotional and/or stress eating.

Some of the women were inspired by their yoga instructor role models and this inspired them to eat healthier. Many individuals studied also felt a sense of acceptance, kindness, and support in the yoga community and this motivated participants to be kinder to themselves in terms of self-care and to not be overly hard on themselves after making less-than-desirable food choices. [1]

95 percent of the individuals said that psychological or mental changes resulted from practicing. In some instances, these changes incited weight loss. Changes mentioned most often were increased mindfulness, clarity, focus, and discipline. Some participants reported improved mood, emotional stability, and reduced reactivity. Others said that as their focus shifted away from weight loss to healthier lifestyles, weight loss became easier.

Overweight participants often said improved self-confidence and self-esteem contributed to their weight loss. They also said their weight loss experiences were markedly different than past attempts. The subjects found losing weight to be easier and felt more confident that they could keep the weight off. [1]

Another study followed 15 women and 2 men practicing Ayurveda and a yoga-based lifestyle at the University of Arizona in Tucson for three months. Weight loss of 3.5 kilograms (7.7 pounds) postintervention and 5.9 kilograms (8.6 pounds) during a follow-up appointment shows evidence that this lifestyle offers promise for sustainable weight loss and lifestyle changes.

Participants reported increased vitality, psychosocial well-being, enhanced quality-of-life and positive adjustments in self-awareness and relationships. [2]

Practicing yoga philosophy, including the Eight Limbs of Yoga, which focus on ethical practices such as non-harm and honesty, may trigger changes in consciousness that lead to better balanced eating. Some yoga poses or asanas facilitate weight loss in different ways. Poses involving twisting of the torso help digestion, standing poses strengthen the large muscles of the thighs, and forward bends stimulate abdominal organs and the thyroid gland. [3]

A public health study of 15,550 adults ages 53 to 57 tracked physical activity (including yoga) and weight change over several years. Practicing yoga for four or more years resulted in reduced age-related weight loss, especially in those who were overweight, compared to the normal population. Scientists concluded that regular yoga practice can help people of all ages lose or maintain body weight. [4]

Yoga is often incorporated into programs for eating disorders and weight management. Obese women who practiced yoga for 16 weeks significantly decreased body weight, body fat percentage, BMI, waist circumference, and visceral fat area compared with a non-exercising group. [5]

A different group of researchers reviewed 20 personal journeys of obese women with binge eating disorders throughout their 12-week yoga treatment program. The women's perspectives on eating improved over the course of the program.

Women reported improved physical self-empowerment, a healthy reconnection with food habits, and cultivated awareness of self and the present moment. Participants ate less, ate slower, and chose healthier foods during the treatment program. The women reported feeling more connected with and positive about their bodies, which translated to better eating habits. [6]

Meditation is another mindful practice that can help you on your healthy lifestyle journey. With eyes closed and breathing relaxed, a person focuses on a thought, object or activity to keep thoughts on the present moment and achieve a calm and stable state of mind. An individual practicing meditation may listen to quiet music, a calming background sound, such as rushing water, and/or follow a guided script during the practice.

People often discount meditation for weight loss since it doesn't burn calories. "Our body is a mirror reflection of what's going on in our minds," writes Dina Kaplan in her 2018 *Forbes* article about meditation and weight loss. "If our primary focus is on losing weight, we cut ourselves off from the emotional and mental beings we are, and that prevents us from understanding why the weight is showing up in the first place."

Kaplan, who started The Path—a company offering meditation classes and retreats—says her clients learn to understand themselves by doing "inner work" including meditation and that helps them to "dig up emotional triggers and past traumas that have manifested into an unhealthy weight and/or relationship with food."

When you better understand yourself, it becomes clear why you skip morning workouts or grab fast food even though you know it's harmful to your health, Kaplan said. "You can explore your motivations for weight loss and why you haven't accomplished your goals." [7]

Yoga Nidra, also known as yogic sleep, is a form of guided meditation where you descend into a deep state of relaxation but are still awake and aware. Some practitioners report one hour of Yoga Nidra being as restorative to the mind and body as two hours of sleep.

Early in the practice, you set a sankalpa or a solemn vow or goal. Your sankalpa should be in the present tense—as if you have already achieved it (such as I am peaceful, I am healthy, I am emotionally balanced...)—and this same vow is best maintained during future practices until you feel that you have reached your objective.

Often these guided meditations have a certain purpose in mind such as sleep, relaxation, or improved awareness. I took an excellent three-day Yoga Nidra workshop in 2018 from Anna Laurita, owner of Davannayoga in Puerto Vallarta, Mexico.

Breathwork, which intentionally changes and manipulates the breath for a period of time, can help people new to meditation and breathing become more comfortable. By focusing on a particular aspect — the sound, the length of the breath, the flow of the breath and other aspects, it is easier to stay in the present moment. Two books I use as resources for breathwork are *Essential Pranayama, Breathing Techniques for Balance, Healing, and Peace* and *Yoga for Pain Relief: Simple Practices to Calm Your Mind and Heal Your Chronic Pain.* [8, 9]

Many apps offer guided meditations or timed meditation sessions. My personal favorite is Insight Timer. I especially enjoy Yoga Nidra sessions by Calgary instructor Tanis Fishman and Soraya Saraswati (yoga therapist and meditation teacher) /Terry Oldfield (musician). Oldfield has created many relaxing songs that I downloaded for yoga practice and meditation.

Practicing yoga, breathwork, and meditation can help you escape the frustrating cycle of yo-yo dieting and demoralizing defeat after weight is regained. You will soon feel more relaxed and likely find that mindful practice will improve many other areas of your life beyond healthier eating habits and reduced hip and waist measurements.

There are many apps you can use for meditation. Headspace, Calm, and Insight Timer are some examples. I like that Insight Timer allows you to do your own timed meditations with your choice of background sounds. You can also set a sound (such as a singing bowl ding) to go off at different intervals that signal how far you are along. This app also offers hundreds of guided meditations.

It will take some work to find the right yoga class. Research what studios are near you and make sure that the instructors are certified by the Yoga Alliance and have taught for at least one year. Yoga Alliance instructors have all had a minimum of 200 hours of training on anatomy and physiology, yoga philosophy, class structures, cueing, and much more.

A gentle or restorative practice is a good choice for starting out. Both practices are great whenever you need to relax. Once you feel comfortable with your practice, you can expand your repertoire of classes.

Different teachers offer styles that appeal to certain individuals. Some instructors cue very well on form and help people individually. Others discuss the chakras (energy centers) and share other aspects of yoga philosophy (which may or may not appeal to you). Your best bet is to sample different classes until you find the right instructor.

Many facilities will offer you a trial membership or even some free classes so you can make sure the studio—and the instructors—are right for you.

Some people feel more comfortable practicing at home. Since the pandemic, I have continued to teach classes on Zoom. I also have a Vimeo page, with hundreds of videos available to stream or download. My videos aren't super high quality (they are recordings of Zoom classes) but they are ideal for older adults with limitations or that are new to yoga. I cue a lot for safety and don't ask participants to do advanced asanas such as headstands and arm balancing poses. A monthly membership giving you access to all of these is only $12.99. The website address where you can find them is https://vimeo.com/ondemand/yogawithsusan

You can also download apps such as Glo and Yoga Anytime, which offer memberships and access to videos.

REFERENCES

1 – Ross, A., A. Brooks, K. Touchton-Leonard, and G. Wallen. 2016. "A Different Weight Loss Experience: A Qualitative Study Exploring the Behavioral, Physical, and Psychosocial Changes Associated with Yoga That Promote

Weight Loss." *Evid Based Complement Alternat Med.* 2016: 2914745.

2 – Rioux, J.; and A. Howerter. 2019. "Outcomes from a Whole-Systems Ayurvedic Medicine and Yoga Therapy Treatment for Obesity Pilot Study." *J Altern Complement Med.* 25(1): S124-S137.

3 – Van Pelt, J. 2012. "Drop Those Pounds With Yoga: Studies Show Yoga Stimulates Weight Loss." *Today's Dietician.* 13(3):18.

4 - Kristal A.R., A. J. Littman, D. Benitez, and E. White. 2005. "Yoga practice is associated with attenuated weight gain in healthy, middle-aged men and women." *Altern Ther Health Med.* 11(4):28-33.

5 - Lee J, J. Kim, and D. Kim. 2011."Effects of yoga exercise on serum adiponectin and metabolic syndrome factors in obese postmenopausal women." *Menopause.* 19(3):296-301.

6 - McIver S., M. McGartland, and P. O'Halloran. 2009. "Overeating is not about the food: women describe their experience of a yoga treatment program for binge eating." *Qual Health Res.* 19(9):1234-1245.

7 - Kaplan, D. 2018. "Here's How Meditation Helps with Weight Loss." *Forbes.* https://www.forbes.com/sites/dinakaplan/2018/01/28/meditation-for-weight-loss-and-holistic-health/?sh=1f58e47bef25

8 - Givens, J. 2020. *Essential Pranayama: Breathing Techniques for Balance, Healing, and Peace.* Emeryville, CA: Rockridge Press.

9 - McGonigal, K. 2009. *Yoga for Pain Relief: Simple Practices to Calm Your Mind and Heal Your Chronic Pain.* Oakland, CA: New Harbinger Publications.

CHAPTER THIRTEEN
Medication-Related Weight Gain

By the time we reach our 50s, many of us are taking daily medications. Every pill you take has a long list of side-effects. In some cases, weight gain is one of them. Although physicians tend to downplay these, medication side-effects are life altering (and not in a good way) for many individuals.

Let's discuss this common problem, why it happens, and how you might be able to remediate the damage.

Some medical conditions, including Polycystic Ovary Syndrome and hypothyroidism, can cause weight to spike. This weight gain usually normalizes with treatment of the disease.

Before you start taking new medications, it is always a good idea to discuss the possible side-effects with your physician. If weight gain is one of them and this concerns you, you might try asking if there is a possibility you could take a lower dose or a different medication.

Here is a list of common medications that have been linked to weight gain.

1 – Tricyclic Antidepressants. Amitriptyline, doxepin, and nortriptyline may increase appetite, causing weight gain. Other classes of antidepressants, including bupropion and duloxetine are associated with weight loss. Fluoxetine is not associated with any weight changes.

2- Corticosteroids. Oral steroids such as prednisone can increase appetite, fluid retention, and may slow your metabolism. Often, they are only prescribed for a week or two. When they are required for chronic conditions, patients will have to be extra mindful about diet and exercise in order to control weight gain.

3 – Antihistamines. Research published in *Obesity* established that people who take antihistamines regularly (Zyrtec, Allegra, Clarinex) have a higher body weight and waist circumference compared to those who don't take them. Histamines in the body turn off hunger signals. Antihistamines may interfere with fullness signals. Nasal steroid sprays such as Flonase, which is not associated with weight gain, may be an option for some individuals.

4 – Epilepsy medications for seizures such as gabapentin, pregabalin, and vigabatrin sometimes increase

appetite and can lead to weight gain. You might talk to your doctor and request a medication associated with weight loss or no gain such as felbamate, topiramate, or lamotrigine.

5 – Beta Blockers used to treat hypertension (Tenormin, metoprolol) may cause weight gain. Doctors believe that the link lies with the fatigue and lack of exercise tolerance that many patients experience. A 2017 study in *Gastroenterology* indicates that the drug may slow metabolism. These medications in general are not recommended for overweight and obese individuals. Consult with your physician to see if ACE inhibitors are a viable option for you.

6 – SSRIs or selective serotonin reuptake inhibitors increase serotonin in the brain, usually to treat depression. Escitalopram, paroxetine, and sertraline may cause weight gain due to increased appetite. Other individuals report weight loss due to improved mood.

7- MAOI or monoamine oxidase inhibitors are used to treat depression or alleviate migraine symptoms. These drugs, particularly phenelzine, may stimulate appetite.

8 – Insulin, used to treat diabetes, may promote weight gain, whenever sugar is not utilized by your body for energy and is directed into fat storage. High sugar foods, such as candy and desserts, will make you more vulnerable to weight gain when you take insulin. Patients with type 1 diabetes must take insulin to keep blood sugar balanced and

remain well. Patients with type 2 diabetes often can make lifestyle changes (improved diet, more exercise) and taper off and eventually eliminate taking insulin (when doctor recommends).

9 – Sulfonylureas (glicylazide, glibenclamide), also used to treat diabetes causes an average weight gain of 4 or 5 pounds. Weight gain occurs as excess sugar ends up converted to fat cells. Ask your doctor about drugs that are weight neutral or that tend to incite weight loss (metformin, SGLT2).

10 – Antipsychotic drugs used to treat schizophrenia and bipolar disorder may impair glucose function, increase cholesterol and triglycerides, and put patients at greater risk of developing metabolic syndrome. The medication most likely to cause weight gain is olanzapine. Lurasidone and ziprasidone are less likely to cause an uptick in weight.

Fortunately, there are many instances where an alternative medication can be chosen to reduce the chance of weight gain. If this option isn't possible, many of the tips I've offered in this book—such as choosing healthy foods, drinking plenty of water, managing stress with mindful practices, and not shopping when you're hungry—will help you to avoid or minimize weight gain from medications.

REFERENCES

1 – Migala, J. 2020. "10 Common Medications That May Cause Weight Gain." *Everyday Health online.* https://www.everydayhealth.com/diet-nutrition/common-medications-that-may-cause-weight-gain/

2 – Ratliff, J., J. Barber, L. Palmese, E. Reutenauer, and C. Tek. 2010. "Association of prescription H1 antihistamine use with obesity: Results from the National Health and Nutrition Examination Survey." *Obesity (Silver Spring).* 18(12): 2398-2400.

3- Igel, L., R. Kumar, K. Saunders, and L. Aronne. 2017. "Practical Use of Pharmacotherapy for Obesity." *Gastroenterology.* 152 (7): 1765-1779.

CHAPTER FOURTEEN

Susan's Slim For Life Secrets

Below are 25 Slim for Life Secrets that will help you on your journey. Many of these have helped me and dozens of friends, family members, and personal training clients to remain at their optimal weight as years pass.

Slim for Life Secret #1 - Avoid Binges at Parties

Curbing snack attacks and warding off the temptation to overeat at parties can be challenging. A small pre-event snack can stabilize blood sugar, keep energy levels high, and prevent intense hunger that can lead to binge eating. Increasing fat intake at meals can reduce hunger and may eliminate uncomfortable hunger or the need for snacks altogether.

The best snacks are filling and packed with nutrients. The worst ones are simple carbohydrates such as candy and pastries loaded with white sugar or corn syrup. Such treats give you a temporary blood sugar high followed by a sudden plummet, which lingers until you pop more sugar in your mouth.

Some of my favorite healthy snacks are small slices of cheese, a dozen nuts (almonds, pistachios or pecans are my favorites), and plain yogurt. You might have to experiment to see which snacks best help you get through vulnerable situations without a binge. Since I no longer snack and I avoid sugar (which always caused my worst cravings), binge eating for me has become a thing of the past.

Eating a small, filling snack ahead of time will allow you to make wiser food choices once you get to the party. Walk by the food table and decide what you're going to put on your plate first. Then get in line and serve yourself what you planned to eat. Savor your food. Once you finish, get rid of your plate and talk to people some distance away from the food so you're not tempted to nibble.

Aim to drink in moderation. Alcoholic beverages are empty calories, which deplete rather than nourish your body. They also reduce inhibitions, leading to overeating. If you must drink, alternate back and forth between your alcoholic beverage and club soda to reduce calorie consumption and the effects of the alcohol on your will power.

Stand, fidget and dance. These "activities" burn calories. Standing burns more calories than sitting. A survey of career women established that those who sat for 361 minutes or more during an average workday were 1.7 times more likely to be overweight than those who sat for 30 minutes or less. [1] Whether you're working or retired, aim to stay on your feet as much as possible. Sitting for long periods of time isn't just a diet buster: it has been linked to many health problems.

If possible, find an ally at the party who wants to employ similar mindful eating strategies. Then you can bond together and "just say no" each time the caterer waves yet another tempting tray in front of your nose.

When hosting a party, serve plenty of healthy, low-fat, low-calorie foods. Vegetable trays with low-fat dressing, fruit trays, cheese trays, and whole grain breadsticks are great options. Many of your guests will appreciate your efforts to provide healthy foods.

REFERENCES

1 - Halvorson, R. 2015. "Frequent Sitting Means Weight Gain for Women." *IDEA Fitness Journal*. 12(3).

Slim for Life Secret #2 - Travel (for Work or Pleasure) Without Gaining Weight

Sixteen years ago, while employed as a sales manager for an assistive technology company, I traveled to conferences and schools in many different states. Diet and exercise became a challenge, but within weeks, I had formulated a strategy. I found ways to exercise daily (even if in small bouts) and avoid sugar-laden breakfasts and unhealthy restaurants.

Aim to find hotels with gyms or near a place (indoor or outdoor) where you can work out. Some hotels offer strength training tools you can check out to use in your room such as dumbbells or stability balls. One tool I highly recommend for travel is the TRX suspension trainer. It is great for strengthening major muscle groups as well as your core. If you're traveling overseas, you'll be able to use it any place you have a door!

Go to https://store.trxtraining.com/shop/suspension-trainers/ to order a TRX trainer. I have written many articles with descriptions and photos of TRX exercises. Most of these are listed on the publication page of my fit women rock website http://fitwomenrock.com/?page_id=392

When traveling for work, I soon learned that restaurant meals posed the biggest threat to my plan to avoid weight gain. I worked hard to ward off the potential damage. The good news is that it's much easier to eat healthy on the run today than it was fifteen years ago. Many fast or to-go style restaurants now offer very healthy and/or low-calorie fare; you just have to choose wisely.

To keep my eating in check, I traveled with oatmeal packets, nuts, and tea bags. That way, I could breakfast in my hotel room, have more time to exercise, and leave feeling satisfied and ready to work. Eating ahead of time kept me from being tempted by doughnuts and sweet rolls, the usual "breakfast" offered at most of the conferences. A breakfast high in simple carbohydrates is not only a disaster for steady blood sugar and energy levels, it also drags you down even more when you're traveling and changing time zones.

I went for salads (dressing on the side), soups (tend to fill me up more than other foods), lunch-sized portions, and heart-healthy meals as often as possible. I sought restaurants offering lunch sized portions at dinner and ordered nutritious meals relatively low in calories (salads packed with fresh veggies and cheese — not loaded with processed meat — with dressing on the side); salmon or other fish filets - grilled or poached, not fried and served with vegetables; grilled chicken, and some Asian and Mediterranean dishes).

I recommend searching for restaurant menus online before dining. Decide what you will order ahead of time based on calories and other nutritional information. I still do this often when I'm about to go out. This way you won't be tempted to order something with twice the calories while you're engaged in conversation or aren't feeling disciplined enough to make a thoughtful choice.

In my *Fitter Than Ever at 40 and Beyond* book, I included a top 10 *Health* article list of the healthiest fast food restaurants. The link to that list is no longer online. I found another one but found it less than impressive. Foods in general weren't healthy and seemed very high in calories.

For that reason, I decided to compile my own list based on my own experience and viewing different fast food menus. I am not going to rank them but I will offer my honest opinion on strengths and weaknesses.

Chipotle Mexican Grill specializes in tacos and burritos—a great option if you love healthy Mexican food. They also offer salads and quesadillas. This restaurant is one of my go-to places after swim meets. I find the portions too large, but the food is super delicious.

The company buys mostly organic produce that is locally purchased and hormone- and antibiotic-free meats. Vegan and vegetarian options are also available and if you eat gluten free you can eat your burrito contents from a bowl, instead of wrapped in a tortilla (burrito bowl). Adding cheese and sour cream can up the calories quickly. Calories of different combos can be calculated at https://chipotle.com/nutrition-calculator

Another favorite of mine is In-N-Out Burger. We always stop at a Tucson location when we return from Mexico and don't have any food in the fridge. Since I don't eat gluten, I order the double-double cheeseburger, protein style (520 calories). The burger is wrapped in lettuce (and a thin layer of paper to make it easier to eat) instead of coming with a bun.

The hamburger is 100 percent USDA ground chuck, free of additives, fillers or preservatives. French fries are made with fresh potatoes (I've seen them dicing them in their machines) and shakes with real ice cream. The burgers and fries are all high in sodium. They have a very simple menu without a lot of elaborate, calorie laden options—a big benefit. Their menu with nutritional information can be found here https://www.in-n-out.com/menu/nutrition-info

Subway is a good lunch-on-the-go option to control calories if you're able to stick to eating a 6-inch sub. Bread is made fresh daily. Comprehensive nutrition information can be viewed at https://www.subway.com/en-US/MenuNutrition/Nutrition/NutritionGrid It was unclear to me on this nutrition page if calories listed are for 6- or 12-inch subs. I cut out processed meats (which increase cancer risk and are high in additives, including MSG), so I no longer buy sandwiches from this chain.

Wendy's is the third-largest hamburger fast food chain in the world. Their buns are loaded with preservatives. Burgers and fries are high in sodium. They do offer some nutritious salads. Check out the salad menu at https://order.wendys.com/category/102/freshmade-salads We often look for these when on the road since they're fairly easy to find.

With a proliferation of sushi restaurants in the US, most people can grab sushi in their neighborhood or wherever they're vacationing. Sushi is basically a seaweed wrap, usually with fish and rice inside and with soy sauce, pickled ginger and wasabi handy to add for flavor. For many years, we dined in a neighborhood sushi restaurant almost every Friday.

Sushi is low in fat. Fish is rich in protein and loaded with heart healthy Omega-3 fatty acids. Sushi restaurants often serve other options that aren't so healthy (very high in saturated fat and sodium) and would be best to pass on, such as teriyaki bowls and fried noodles. Sushi made with raw fish does put you at risk for infection from bacteria or parasites. It is safer to opt for vegetarian sushi or sushi made with cooked fish.

Fast food places I tend to avoid are McDonald's, Arby's, Taco Bell, and Long John Silver's. In general, I recommend that you avoid places that offer super caloric foods you can't resist, that have no healthy options, or that don't list calories on their menu pages.

When traveling, especially for an extended time, your diet choices are critical. It's easy to swallow 1500 to 2000 calories in one poorly chosen restaurant meal. If you make good food choices, burning calories with exercise can be a second way to mitigate weight gain when traveling. Regular activity can also help manage stress, which is a common trigger for eating binges.

Here's what I did to stay active during my work-related trips:

1 - I chose hotels with gyms and pools (and checked to make sure they were open during the hours I could use them). Some hotels also offer free use of nearby fitness facilities. This can be great if they're conveniently located.

2 - I awoke early every morning to exercise. Since I was on my feet most of the day, I chose swimming or stationary bicycling for aerobic exercise. I only had time for about 30 minutes of exercise daily, but I was able to also fit in other short bursts of activity. If you're going to be sitting most of the day, the treadmill and/or the elliptical will be good choices if no physical limitations make those activities prohibitive.

3 - I walked whenever possible — up and down the hall or around the parking lot or block during lunches and

breaks between meetings and around the airport terminal when waiting for flights. I took the stairs to get to my hotel room when I had an upper level floor. Any time you can insert a few minutes of activity, do so!

4 - I put a resistance band around my ankles when getting ready in the morning. Moving around the room like this with the bands helped tone my thighs and buttocks.

When planning leisure travel, I often dive into activities I don't normally do at home. I swim in a new body of water (ocean or lake), do yoga (outdoors, of course), rent an e-bike, and take long hikes or walks. Sometimes, we embark on activity-based vacations.

So far, my husband and I have gone scuba diving in Mexico, Belize, Jamaica, the Bahamas, and Costa Rica, cycled through the Swiss Alps, hiked to Machu Picchu, circumnavigated several Greek Islands in the Ionian Sea, and hiked to many Mayan Ruins in Belize and Guatemala. All these trips were delightful fun. While staying active all day, we met interesting people from around the world and enjoyed beautiful views and plenty of fresh air! What could be better?

REFERENCES

1 - Cox, L. 2012. "Why is Too Much Salt Bad for You?" *Live Science online* (http://www.livescience.com/36256-salt-bad-health.html)

Susan's Slim for Life Secret #3 -Minimize Restaurant Meals

It's understandable that you might need to eat out often when you're traveling, but what do you do at home? If you're dining out often, please reconsider this habit. It will greatly simplify and ease your journey to wellness.

Did you know that many restaurant meals are packed with 2000 or more calories? It's true. And that's just for the appetizer, soup or salad, main course, and dessert. That doesn't even include your glass or two of wine or the fancy cocktail you decide to order.

In a book entitled, *So You're Fat. Now What?* cardiologist Salvatore Tirrito says, "I will go as far to say that if you eat out more than twice a week, you are probably never going to lose any weight."

Honestly, his assessment corresponds with what I've observed after more than thirty years on the ground training and teaching fitness. I never trained a client who wanted to lose weight, ate out more than three times a week and reached their weight loss goal. It is like trying to swim upstream in a heavy current!

I suggest you save yourself the needless frustration. Until you reach your goal weight, please keep meals out to a minimum and when you do eat out, choose restaurants that list calories of menu items and that serve smaller portions. Eating in restaurants these days essentially teaches you to not be satisfied until you've finished enormous quantities of food!

Do you want to know how many calories (and how much saturated fat, etc.) you consume when you eat out? Go to restaurant websites to learn the ugly truth. Many of these links change often, so if you get a dead link, go to the main website and then hunt around.

Some sites only have nutrition listed if you click a link next to each item; others have a page that lists nutritional information on all available items. I have decided not to list links in this book since the menus and links change so often. It's easy enough to search on your phone before you go. If a restaurant doesn't share nutritional information, it's best to stay away.

These snacks and meals can really blow your diet…

- Starbucks Grande Café Vanilla Frappuccino with blueberry muffin **910 calories**
- Pizza Hut personal pan cheese pizza and 16-oz. Coke **830 calories**
- Ben and Jerry's Chunky Monkey (1 pint) **1160 calories**
- Schlotzsky's Deli Original Sandwich and 16-oz Coke **975 calories**
- Big Mac, medium fries and chocolate shake at McDonald's **1470 calories**

Any time nutrition information isn't available, assume you are getting 600 calories from each appetizer, 400 for a soup or salad, 1000 for a main course and 600 for a dessert.[1]

Can you say "Ouch?" Are you still too speechless? Let me say it for you—"Ouch!" If you study restaurant menus too long, you might need to have the paramedics standing by. The shock factor is so extreme.

The quickest way to resuscitate your diet is to take control and eat more meals at home. I intentionally minimize meals out for better health and weight control. I like to have control over what I'm eating and to avoid foods with added sugar or transfat. I can consume fewer calories and healthier meals eating at home and save a lot of money, too.

REFERENCES

1 - Tirrito, S. 2009. *So You're Fat. Now What?* Wheatmark.

Susan's Slim for Life Secret # 4 - Avoid Artificial Sweeteners

Consuming foods and beverages with artificial sweeteners might seem like the perfect way to kick your weight loss plan into high gear. They contain fewer calories than sugar-laden drinks and will lead to weight loss, right? Think again. The research shows just the opposite. People who consume artificial sweeteners tend to weigh more than those who turn their noses up at them.

Read your labels. Drinks and foods containing aspartame will not only sabotage your weight loss efforts, they may also sabotage your health. Aspartame, made by joining the amino acids aspartic acid and phenylalanine, although declared safe by many certifying agencies, possibly negatively impacts health. It is purportedly 200 times as sweet as sugar, meaning you could use a much smaller quantity and still be satisfied, which once again sounds good, but isn't so great when you dig deeper.

Many studies indicate consuming artificial sweeteners correlates with weight gain. For some reason, rats and people consuming artificial sweeteners ate up to four times as much as people and rats eating only foods sweetened with regular sugar! It appears that consuming artificial sweeteners interferes somehow with the body's natural ability to regulate calorie intake.

A study following thousands of residents of San Antonio for 10 years found those who drank more than 21 servings of diet drinks a week were at twice the risk of becoming overweight or obese, and the more diet soda people drank, the greater the risk.[1]

I'll add some anecdotal evidence to this mix. During the only time in my life where I experienced weight problems, I drank two or three diet sodas per day. I look back and remember how I felt constantly hungry and deprived. I even dreamed about fattening food at night! Somehow, artificial sweeteners had the same effect on my body as real sweeteners.

The more I consumed the more I ate overall throughout the day. This still holds true for me with foods high in sugar (I now also avoid artificial sweeteners like the plague). When I start eating sweets, I notice I eat up to 20 percent more throughout the day and constantly feel hungry. That's why I rarely eat them.

Sucralose, used in many beverages and even yogurt, is another commonly used artificial sweetener with questionable consequences on weight and health. I suggest you ditch the diet sodas and the "sugar-free" junk food and pour yourself a glass of water with a little lemon instead.

REFERENCES

1 - Rabin, R. 2016. "Artificial Sweeteners and Weight Gain." *New York Times Blog*. https://well.blogs.nytimes.com/2016/02/19/artificial-sweeteners-and-weight-gain/

Susan's Slim for Life Secret # 5 - Avoid Fake Food

If you've ever read food labels, you'll notice that many items contain more than 10 ingredients. Those "fresh" baked items from the grocery store may contain 25 or 30 ingredients, including many preservatives—so the bread or pastry can stay on the shelf longer without spoiling—and colorants to make the food look good so it will lure you to buy it. Often some unhealthy oils thrown into the mix.

A Dairy Queen chocolate ice cream cone contains 22 ingredients. Many Americans consume five pounds of additives per year.[1] Yuck! I read labels like that and think that item doesn't sound at all like food to me! And I don't buy it.

One of the big risks of eating preservative-rich foods is that many are classified as hyperpalatable. What this means is that food companies have designed them to tap into your brain's reward system, predisposing you and all the rest of us to have an addictive-like craving for them.

If we eat enough of these foods, eventually whole foods (that are not processed at all or that are minimally processed) will begin to taste bland and inedible and only unhealthy foods packed with salt, sugar, and/or fat will do. Once addictive behavior takes hold, it is much harder for a person to eat to sate hunger instead of giving into emotional cravings.[3]

Lab rats given unlimited access to a diet high in carbohydrates and fat will nearly eat themselves to death and will walk across an electrified plate to get to their junk food. Once addicted to all three substances, when given a choice between sugar, cocaine and alcohol, the rats ran straight for the sugar.[4]

If you have been suffering under a shroud of guilt, thinking that it's your fault that you have no will power to stop eating this stuff, recognize that food companies are manipulating minds (and tastebuds) so almost no one who eats this stuff can say *no*. The only way to free yourself is to stop eating this addictive food.

When you constantly indulge in foods rich in sugar and fat, overeating and addiction becomes part of your gene expression.[4] Altering your genetic "story" starts that first day you choose to eat an apple instead of a candy bar.

I'm very familiar with food addiction because I suffered from it for years. There were times where the only thing that mattered was sinking my teeth into a pizza with melted cheese or getting my hands on that bag of vending machine chocolates (that had fallen from the hook and gotten stuck on the way down)!

I wouldn't have cared if our dormitory roof collapsed or the fire alarm went off. My hands literally trembled when I was in line waiting to buy junk food at a convenience store. From my experience, the only path to freedom is to wean yourself off of these foods. They wreak havoc on your weight, your self-esteem and your health.

No one really knows the long-term effects of eating a preservative-rich diet. I have read studies that show that if certain food particles, such as the artificial sweetener sucralose, are not recognized by the digestive system, they may remain in your gut.[1] Some preservatives upset the natural balance of intestinal flora. Is there any wonder most

Americans never leave home without several different products for upset stomachs and bowel issues?

If you experience headaches or other symptoms from MSG, be aware that more than 40 different items with different names also contain this harmful substance including seemingly benign items such as gelatin and whey protein.[2] "Spices" can include almost anything. That's why when grilling fish or any other meat, I mix up my own blend of healthy spices instead of opting for a pre-made spice mix that is full of questionable ingredients. It only takes a minute.

In general, shop the perimeter of the grocery store. That's where you'll usually find the "real" food. Even then, please read labels like a hawk. I mostly buy fresh (mostly organic) fruits and vegetables, meat, dairy, lentils, quinoa, coffee, and tea. If you've been skimping on produce purchases because of budget, re-evaluate. Do you want to invest money now feeding your body nutritious food to stay healthy or pay it to the hospital later after your body has broken down due to poor nutrition?

Some of my favorite foods are grilled salmon, bonita (a fish my neighbors catch in Mexico), chicken, ribeye, mushrooms sauteed in olive oil, fresh yogurt (I make it myself), berries of any kind (blackberries, blueberries, strawberries, etc.), grapes, nuts (pistachios, pecans, macadamia nuts), spinach, asparagus, avocados, kale, tomatoes, cucumber, broccoli, cheese (swiss, feta, and manchego) and sweet potatoes. Whenever possible, I buy organic.

REFERENCES

1 - Balch, P. 2010. *Prescription for Nutritional Healing Fifth Edition: A Practical A-to-Z Reference to Drug-Free Remedies Using Vitamins, Herbs, and Food Supplements.* New York: Avery (a member of Penguin Group).

2 – Truth In Labeling.
http://www.truthinlabeling.org/hiddensources.html

3 - Parker-Pope, T. 2009. "How the Food Makers Captured Our Brains." *New York Times online.*
(http://www.nytimes.com/2009/06/23/health/23well.html)

4 - Peeke, P. 2012. "The Dopamine Made Me Do it." *IDEA Fitness Journal.* 9(9): 34-42.

Susan's Slim for Life Secret #6 - Ditch Caloric Beverages

When my daughter was in high school, she lost 20 pounds. She didn't go on a starvation diet. She didn't cut out all dairy or eat only soup. She didn't change what she ate at all in fact. She simply stopped drinking juice and soda.

A glass of most liquids other than water or black tea or coffee usually means beaucoup calories. You can drink a whole day's worth of calories inadvertently in a matter of minutes. A single soda contains about 200 calories. That doesn't sound like much, but if you drink three sodas and two glasses of juice during the day, you'll top 1000 calories with drinks alone. Drinking these beverages will also tend to increase, rather than sate your appetite.

Workout or electrolyte drinks, such as Gatorade (127 calories for 16 oz.), that are high in sugar, may compromise dental health. I have had all clean dental checkups since I ditched the habit of drinking sugary energy drinks at work. Low calorie workout drinks tend to be loaded with artificial sweeteners and other chemicals.

I drink water with a dose of salt and magnesium whenever I need electrolytes. A reliable electrolyte supplement you can take after long workouts or exercising in the heat is Hi-Lyte, which offers sodium, potassium and magnesium without any added sugar or chemicals.

Alcoholic beverages can be another caloric black hole. A four-ounce margarita packs about 168 calories, but depending on the size of your drink glass, you might get double or triple the calories. Some drinks excessively high in calories are strawberry daiquiris, piña coladas, and Long Island iced tea (780 calories). I will say that having a beer or glass of wine at parties (when there was a long wait for food) often took the edge off of my appetite and helped me to relax, enabling me to eat less.

I suggest drinking water, unsweetened coffee and tea and having a soda or an alcoholic drink only occasionally. If plain water doesn't please your taste buds, try squeezing in a few drops of lemon juice or adding a tablespoon of coconut water. By dumping the caloric drink habit, you will likely lose weight if you don't subconsciously (or consciously) decide to "reward" yourself with more food.

Susan's Slim for Life Secret #7 - Eat Nutritious, Filling Foods

Many people who reduce caloric intake complain of rabid hunger. It's impossible to lose weight when you're constantly hungry. I know because I've tried it. Oh, I lost a few pounds here and there for a few days. Eventually, being the human I am and disliking the discomfort of a constantly growling stomach, I decided I didn't want to dream about food anymore and obsess about it all day... So, I started eating. And once I started, since I was so starved (enough that I probably would have eaten wallpaper paste if that was all that was available), I ate and ate and ate!

By eating satisfying, filling foods, you can lose weight without suffering from uncomfortable hunger pangs that will inevitably lead to bingeing. Foods high in fat or fiber provide a sense of fullness that lasts. Increasing protein intake can also help with appetite control.

Foods high in sugar will raise and crash your blood sugar and lead you to crave food more often. As I mentioned earlier, I can reduce my food consumption by about 20 percent (easily) by cutting out sweets. A very good friend of mine lost eight pounds in one month simply by eliminating sugar!

I recently started eating yogurt for breakfast most mornings. I add melted butter, fruit, and nuts to balance it out. Yogurt is rich in calcium, B vitamins, and most contain probiotics, which can improve digestive health. Other hunger sating foods that I recommend are oatmeal, Swiss muesli, soups (packed with lentils, quinoa, pinto beans, and/or mung beans), toast with peanut or almond butter, and apples with peanut butter. Baked oatmeal with peaches and blueberries is also delicious. You can check out my recipe in Appendix III.

If you decide to adopt my yogurt habit, don't think that means you have to kiss enjoyment of breakfast goodbye! A yogurt breakfast doesn't have to be boring. Add blueberries, raspberries, mango, flax seed, chia seeds, macadamia nuts, sliced banana, honey, raisins or other dried fruit, and try seasoning with cinnamon or cardamom.

Susan's Slim for Life Secret #8 - Grocery Shop Mindfully

We've all heard the *don't shop when you're hungry* suggestion before, but do you actually follow it? If not, please start today.

Even the most disciplined person's willpower crumbles under the wrong circumstances. If it's been hours since your last meal, pushing the shopping cart past baked goods and tempting smelling foods at the deli without grabbing something (or a few somethings) not on the list will be nearly impossible. Since like you, I'm only human, I've ended up with unintended items as a result of this slip up.

Taking a list will help if you stick to it. Walking only the perimeter of the store is safest—all the junk lurks in the middle aisles. Remember, if the pastries, candy bars, and ice cream never make it to your house, they won't make it to your mouth...or your waistline. One of my biggest strategies for staying away from sweets is never buying them!

I know I mentioned this before, but I'm going to say it again because it's very important. If you don't want to spend time reading labels, please buy items that don't have an ingredient list—fresh food. That makes shopping super easy and doesn't require reading glasses. In the long run, it will improve your health and help you drop unwanted pounds.

Susan's Slim for Life Secret # 9 - Eat Slowly and Without Distraction

Many of us develop the habit of reading, watching TV or working on the computer while eating. Maybe we sit down in front of the TV with a bag of chips only to find when it's over or we're interrupted by an ad or the phone that we've polished off the whole bag! Mindless eating is a habit that is disastrous for your health and waistline.

If you're engaged in some other activity beyond eating, your mind and body don't fully process that you're enjoying a meal. Often the "full" feeling won't come as soon or ever. More than likely, you'll overeat a lot and barely notice. If you're holding a plate of food in your lap while watching TV, you may gobble it down quickly because you're focused on the show plot, not what you're shoveling into your mouth.

Normally, your stomach takes about 10 minutes to give you a signal that you're full but if you eat faster than that, you won't receive a signal in time. And if your mind is somewhere else, you won't ever get one.

Break the doing-something-else-while-eating habit and you'll be able to eat fewer calories at meals without feeling deprived. Savor every bite. Put your fork down often and chew your food well before swallowing. Eating slower and chewing food well enhances digestion.

Susan's Slim for Life Secret #10 - Combat Emotional Eating

During my college days, too much of my eating was "emotional." I'd go out and have way too many drinks for fun and to cope with the stress of college life. After a night out, my friends and I would polish off a large pizza within minutes because the alcohol had loosened our inhibitions. I'd try to go back to dieting and then end up rewarding myself with chips, popcorn and sweets whenever it came time to study for a test or exam.

Feeling distressed over a breakup with a boyfriend or some other issue, I'd reach for more junk food. My diet rollercoaster and these emotional eating habits led to a weight gain of more than 25 pounds. That's quite a lot of weight for my small frame to carry!

I've re-established good eating habits, but it took a lot of hard work to get there. I used to salivate just watching a food commercial on TV. Eating was an emotional reaction instead of a reaction to hunger. I became a food drama queen and allowed my brain to swindle me into believing I had to have food to endure this or that "horrible" period of stress.

My eating today is always hunger-driven. If pangs of hunger or stomach noises make it difficult to keep writing, I'll eat a meal. To keep on a comfortable schedule, I try not to vary my mealtimes by more than an hour.

I never eat just because food is available. When someone offers me food when I'm not hungry, I politely decline. Watching food commercials on TV never propels me toward the refrigerator unless it's close to mealtime. I'm not telling you this to brag. I'm doing this to encourage you. I've already told you enough stories about how far off track I once was to give you evidence that if I can do it, so can you!

Stress can be a major trigger for over-eating and other bad habits such as shopping binges and drug and alcohol abuse. Dopamine, the "feel good" neurotransmitter, tends to be lowest in the late afternoon, making us crave a reward. Low dopamine and serotonin levels often compel people to eat anything in sight (especially foods high in sugar and fat).

This compulsion to eat too much of the wrong foods can be an addiction very similar to a frantic desire for drugs and alcohol.[1] Late afternoon and evenings are times when many of us need to be armed and ready to combat this impulsive

"I have to have it now" hunger with a healthy and satisfying snack.

I used to be really hungry in the late afternoon when I got home from work. This was the time I was most tempted to turn to junk food for a pick me up. I would get home hungry and tired and feel that impulse to turn to food for solace. I used to eat fruit and nuts for snacks most of the time.

Now that I have eliminated snacks, I meditate or read to replenish my energy. I especially enjoy these experiences if weather permits and I'm able to step outside to enjoy them.

In an earlier chapter, I discussed how much yoga and meditation can help you to overcome stress and emotional eating. If you haven't tried it yet, please do. You'll be so pleased with the many benefits you reap from this simple choice.

I have this weird habit of walking by the deli and looking at cakes, doughnuts and pies (when I'm not hungry). Sometimes I even pick up the packages and read the ingredients. And then I smugly set them down and walk away, feeling empowered by the fact that I looked at these items and decided on my own volition to avoid them.

I couldn't have done this 25 years ago (when I constantly ate on impulse), but since I now use hunger as a trigger to eat rather than enticing smells and the sight of appetizing food, it's very easy.

While writing this book, I visited many fast food restaurant websites to find nutrition information (after finishing lunch) and didn't find the photos of burgers and French fries the least bit tempting. I know this sounds crazy, but if you learn to react to real hunger and not impulse on a regular basis it will start to become a habit and no longer a challenge of willpower.

Find ways to manage your stress that don't involve overindulging in comfort food. Take a warm bath, read a good book, meditate, do a Yoga Nidra session, or take a long walk. Even a five-minute time out for some long, restorative breaths will lower your stress level, blood pressure and heart rate.

Once you begin assuaging your stress with non-food pleasures, eating will no longer be the automatic turn-to response when something goes wrong.

REFERENCES

1 - Peeke, P. 2012. "The Dopamine Made Me Do it." *IDEA Fitness Journa*l. 9(9): 34-42.

Susan's Slim for Life Secret #11 - Find Enjoyable Exercise

Most people don't enjoy performing the same exercise day after day. If your cardio consists of walking mindlessly on the treadmill five days a week for an hour, you might soon get to the point where you'd rather go to the dentist and get a root canal than endure yet another boring workout.

If you hate your chosen exercise modality or are bored with it, eventually you will quit. At the minimum, you'll make excuses not to do it. That's why you should take the time early on to seek out exercise you enjoy.

There are so many different modes of activity. Swimming, running, walking, hiking, tennis (and other racquet sports), golf (walking the course), bicycling, stationary gym equipment, kayaking, paddle boarding, rappelling, dance (salsa, merengue, aerobic, ballroom, country, so many others), yoga, Pilates, drumming, and water aerobics.

Spend a month experimenting and then narrow it down to what you like the most, so you keep moving. Most of you will find that mixing it up with two or more activities works best.

Nancy Patchell Knoll, a former SaddleBrooke, Arizona resident and client who followed the *Fitter Than Ever* program, wrote, "As a child, I sat inside reading and did well in school. I did not like playing outside and never played sports like other kids. I barely tolerated required PE courses and did the least possible."

By 2009, Nancy was in her 60s and her lifetime of inactivity was catching up with her. Nancy's doctor urged her to exercise and so she committed to trying my program for six months.

"My BMI and body fat analysis were horrifying. I had worn elastic waist, stretchy pants for decades so I had no idea that I was as big as I measured. I also realized I hadn't looked at myself in a full-length mirror for a long time and was relying on mirrors showing my top half only.

"The first exercise class I took just about killed me in the first 3 minutes. I was having trouble breathing and every muscle in my body hurt—and the class had barely begun. I realized how truly out of shape I was. Everyone told me things would get better as I got into shape, but I was still skeptical."

Jump ahead two months. "As I was able to do more and last longer, I started feeling a sense of pride in myself. An avowed couch potato having fun in aerobics class? Maybe I had changed."

Nancy continued exercising during her summer months away from SaddleBrooke. "I found two new-to-me exercises in Illinois that are social, fun, and great workouts. One is

Nordic walking—I just bought my second set of poles to take back to Arizona. The other is the senior version of Drums Alive, which uses drumming as the exercise. Liking the exercise classes made it so much easier to go. For the first time in my life, exercise is a part of my day and my routine. I make time for it daily. On the few days I can't, it feels weird not to be doing something physical. I just bought two pairs of jeans with zippers and all!"

Consider your personality when you choose exercise modalities and then soon you, like Nancy, will have an exercise success story to tell. Some people really enjoy team activities. Others like to have their exercise be meditative or an outdoor nature experience.

I tend to have days when I want to exercise alone and others where I want to be more social. I take/teach classes some days and do solo walks, kayaks, and swims other days. I love hiking in parks and on beaches where I feel connected to nature. In addition to exercise opportunities, I find these outdoor sessions relaxing and restorative.

Many people find a buddy system improves commitment and motivation to exercise. Your buddy can be someone (or more than one person) you exercise with and/or speak to periodically to provide and ask for encouragement along the way. Having a friend to lean on can be especially helpful when obstacles threaten to derail you from your program.

Most people work harder around others. Perhaps you can run or walk with friends who maintain a similar pace so you can socialize a little and push yourself at the same time.

You could find out about bike rides or running groups in your community so you can meet and connect with others who enjoy the sport. You could swim on a U.S. Masters team (some other countries also have competitive swimming groups and races for adults) and do organized interval workouts instead of slogging out endless boring laps.

You might even be able to find a friend interested in losing weight and getting fitter by doing this program with you. Then you can make appointments to go on a walk, take an exercise class or meet at the gym. Because of the accountability, you'll be less likely to skip workouts and more likely to adhere to the program.

Susan's Slim for Life Secret # 12 - Avoid Over Exercising

You probably thought you would never hear me say don't exercise too much, but here I go...Don't exercise too much! I've done it before, and it only made my battle with weight more difficult. I felt so frustrated and angry that I was running so many miles and hating it and I still wasn't losing weight. It took me a few years to learn why this happens.

Like a starvation diet, extreme levels of activity confuse the body and tend to make it hoard every calorie you eat as if it might be your last. It may also cause your body to release stress hormones, which make it even more difficult to lose weight.

Many studies, including a review that followed *The Biggest Loser* contestants, show that RMR (resting metabolic rate) slows when people follow extreme exercise and diet plans.[1] This makes weight loss and maintenance extremely difficult and frustrating!

I know dozens of overweight athletes who exercise for four or more hours per day and haven't lost weight. If your goal is to do long distance events, engage in a moderate amount of exercise until you achieve your goal weight and then gradually increase duration and intensity. Why not make things easier on yourself rather than as difficult as possible?

The best way to avoid a major decline in RMR is to take a moderate approach to caloric intake and exercise. You will have a much better chance of losing weight if you keep your exercise to 60 to 90 minutes per day. You can burn additional calories by sitting less. Moderate, rather than fanatical, exercise offers the most health benefits anyway. If you want to compete in triathlons, sign up for the minitriathlons (~800 yard swim, ~12 mile bike, 3 mile run), which give you a good balance of a moderate amount of different activities.

REFERENCES

1 - Kolata, G. 2016. "After 'The Biggest Loser' Their Bodies Fought to Regain the Weight." *The Science of Fat.* (NY Times online post) https://www.nytimes.com/2016/05/02/health/biggest-loser-weight-loss.html)

2 – Lee, I.M., L. Djoussé, H.D. Sesso, L. Wang, and J.E. Buring. 2010. "Physical activity and weight gain prevention." *JAMA.* 303(12):1173-1179.

Susan's Slim for Life Secret #13 - Dump the Excuses

You won't succeed at losing weight or changing your habits until you commit to it. There are generally five stages people go through before making major life changes. These are pre-contemplation (not yet ready to change), contemplation (weighing the costs and benefits), preparation (buying a gym membership, hiring a personal trainer), action (exercising, eating healthy), and maintenance (healthy lifestyle has become a habit and is no longer a struggle).[1]

By the time you reach the preparation stage, you need to convince yourself that making excuses will no longer be acceptable.

Most of us conjure up excuses to avoid things we deem unpleasant. I tend to experience a variety of mysterious illnesses the day before dental appointments.

If you followed my previous Slim for Life Secret #10 on enjoyable exercise, hopefully you have now found an activity you look forward to and won't even try to avoid! Hopefully, you've begun trying new food items and have begun to develop a taste for healthier fare.

Long before you picked up this book, you had already made a commitment to certain aspects of your life—non-negotiable responsibilities that you do daily no matter what. If you're employed, you go to work every day unless you're ill or on vacation.

Hopefully, you brush your teeth two or more times a day to maintain your dental health. If you're raising a family, you undoubtedly grocery shop and prepare balanced meals with help from your spouse. You don't make an excuse and say you're not fixing dinner one night, leaving everyone hungry!

You need to consider healthy eating and exercise, like brushing your teeth or fixing your family dinner or going to work or a doctor's appointment, a responsibility, not something you shrug off with an "I don't have time today." Exercise is done at times you pre-schedule. Eating healthy becomes something that you commit time to (buying healthy food items, looking up healthy recipes, and preparing food), not something that you will do again tomorrow or next week or next month. Make healthy living a part of every day instead of making excuses that keep you in a rut. You're worth investing the effort.

Research shows that people tend to eat more when they think about how they'll diet tomorrow or do more exercise in the future. If you have avoided exercise and cutting calories for years, why would you expect it would be any different tomorrow?

Instead of giving yourself the license to head in the wrong direction, go in the right direction while you've got this book in front of you and the will to move forward.

REFERENCES

1 - Prochaska, J.O., J.C. Norcross, and C.C. DiClemente. 1994. *Changing For Good: The Revolutionary Program That Explains The Six Stages Of Change And Teaches You How To Free Yourself From Bad Habits.* New York: W. Morrow.

Susan's Slim for Life Secret #14 - Adopt a New Attitude

Have you ever noticed how when you complain, you feel even worse afterward? I sure have. I do it and then lament the time lost and the fact that I may have pulled someone else's mood down along with mine. Complaining can greatly impair your diet and exercise program results.

I often hear people say, "I'm not sure how much longer I can stand this stupid diet" or "I'm sweating like a pig at the gym every day and for what?" or "I hate to exercise" or "I hate to sweat." This kind of negative chatter—outloud or even allowed to run free inside your mind—gives you close to a zero percent chance of succeeding.

In the August 9, 2009 edition of *TIME*, in an article entitled "Why Exercise Won't Make You Thin," author John Cloud moans that his trainer "will work him like a farm animal, sometimes to the point that I am dizzy." What exactly does this mean? That his trainer collared him, hooked a plow up to him and took him out to till the fields of New York City (do they even have fields there)? And men say that women are drama queens—Ha!

Anyway, back to my original point. If you say, "I hate it," you will hate it. If you say, "I can't do it," you won't succeed. Your mind really does govern your experience.

Here's an experiment you can try, which can give you some perspective on the mental aspect of experience. Frown for 20 minutes. Now pause to notice what kind of mood you are in. Now smile for 20 minutes and see what kind of mood you are in at this point. Now think about a place you really hate for five minutes. How do you feel? And now think of a place that is a peaceful sanctuary for you. Is your mood different? Attitude really is everything.

If you hate to sweat, remind yourself that you are ridding your body of toxins and making your fat cells cry. This is much more positive than whining. Your attitude will have much more influence on whether you succeed at making positive changes than anything else in this book!

If you find a reason to love what you are doing for yourself, eventually it will become a comfortable part of your life. To me, my daily exercise is every bit as comforting to me as my 10-year-old pair of slippers and my afternoon cup of green tea. It is something I can depend on amidst life's many uncertainties.

Some new ways to view this program (and to explain what you are doing to family and friends). "I'll feel so much better after I work out." "This class always helps me manage stress." "I feel empowered making good choices." "I'm making my body healthier." "I feel 20 years younger now that I'm taking better care of myself." "I'm not on a diet. I'm eating healthy foods that give me more energy, keep me satisfied, and taste better the more often I eat them."

Susan's Slim for Life Secret #15 - Live Young

When a woman's attitude ages, she may convince herself that she is too old to [fill in the blank] — watch what she eats, compete in athletic events, spend time exercising, wear shorts, bathing suits, bike pants and/or Spandex, or swim. And for that reason, she stops doing these things and before long the appearance of her body starts to match her mindset.

Just say "no" to that confining realm of thinking old. Go ahead and buy the neon-colored tights or the thong bathing suit. And when your daughter asks you if you'd like to give her extra paddleboard a try, don the safety vest, grab a paddle and head out with her on a new adventure!

Before I met my husband and used a dating service, I met a man who left a recording in my voicemail box saying he enjoyed cycling, hiking, rock climbing and scuba diving. I looked forward to meeting him and imagined all the outdoor adventures we would enjoy together.

When I met him, he confessed that he no longer did those activities. Now he was tired and busy with work and starting to have aches and pains. He was only in his mid 30s! Needless to say, that connection didn't last long. I find it exhausting to spend time with people who act and think old. When I encountered them as clients, I tried to help them reframe their thinking so they could enjoy life more!

If you've given up activities you love for committees, shopping trips, TV, knitting, and other activities you somehow deem age appropriate, I suggest you reevaluate your priorities and mentally turn back the clock. If you're doing exercise that "people your age do," rebel and try something fun instead. When was the last time you saw a child on a treadmill?

Just because you're over fifty doesn't mean you shouldn't have fun being active! If you love riding a unicycle (and have good bone density and excellent balance), go buy one. If you once loved trampolining (I do), purchase a big one or a mini-tramp, but make sure there are spotters all around you or that you have a safety net (or bar for the mini-tramp).

Do you like horseback riding? Find a facility with well-trained horses where you can embark on a guided trail ride. Reclaim your youthful perspective on exercise and you'll find it so much easier to be active.

I've studied the habits of many very fit older adults and their workout schedules and attire closely resemble those of people half their age. They don't use their age as an excuse to be sedentary or to justify carrying around excess weight.

They're not embarrassed to wear a swimsuit because of droopy skin or a few wrinkles. They continue to live the active lives they've always lived. For me, the title of Olympic swimmer Dara Torres' book *Age is Just a Number* says it all. Shrug your shoulders and keep moving and you'll look a whole lot better than if you start telling yourself you're too old to do this or that anymore.

In 2008, I interviewed 90-year-old Rita Simonton, who set several world records for 90-94-year-old women at the U.S. Masters Long Course Swimming Nationals event in Portland, Oregon. When I punched in her number and waited for her to answer, I worried that she might be easily confused or have trouble hearing. Instead, she was enthusiastic and quick-witted. Within minutes, I nearly forgot I was speaking to someone twice my age. She quickly showed her mind to be as agile as her body.

When training clients at SaddleBrooke, an active adult community in northwest Tucson, I saw the same familiar faces nearly every morning. Women in their 50s, 60s and even their 90s, clad in running shorts, Spandex bottoms, and/or tank tops that showed-off well-toned muscles. They do Zumba classes, high intensity interval training (HIIT) workouts, strength training workouts, or core work and then head out to play tennis or golf. Some are on the community swimming team or members of the cycling or the hiking club. None of these people would say they are too old to go cycling or wear shorts or a form-fitting top.

One couple in their 80s came to the gym three times a week (in their cycling shorts after a ride) to do their weight workouts together. Nancy always stood out from the crowd in her bright red cycling shorts! I remember how they always took turns spotting each other on the bench press machine. There's something about seeing couples support each other in their training efforts that always warms my heart.

In Mexico, I have a friend in her mid-70s who mountain bikes for two to three hours more than once a week. She broke a forearm bone once, but that didn't stop her from getting back to it once the doctor cleared her to! Mountain biking is what she enjoys most and so she continues to pursue it with passion!

Many other friends and neighbors in their 70s are out kayaking with the dolphins most days of the week (there are "peddle" kayaks available on the market today that don't require upper body strength and work better for people with previous shoulder issues). My neighbors recently bought stair-stepper style paddleboards that look like a lot of fun.

Stock up on shoes and other athletic wear that you will need to move comfortably as you begin exercising. Consider leaving the gray and black workout wear on the rack and step out in something bright and flashy that you imagine area high school kids would envy. If it makes you feel excited about what you are about to do, why not go for it?

Slim for Life Secret #16 - Drink Before You Eat

Most of us have heard that old adage drink water before each meal. That's a good tip to remember anytime you feel hungry. Sometimes signals get crossed and you feel hungry when you're really dehydrated. When a snack attack strikes, drink a glass of water before opening the refrigerator. Often the water will give you a sense of fullness and you'll consume less food as a result.

Consuming water improves digestion and increases metabolism.[2] Always drink a glass of water before your breakfast, lunch and dinner. A study showed that dieters drinking 500 ml of water (16.9 ounces) before meals experienced more weight loss than the people restricting calorie consumption who didn't consume the pre-meal water. [1]

REFERENCES

1 - Dennis E.A., A.L. Dengo, D.L. Comber, K.D. Flack, J. Savla, K.P. Davy, and B.M. Davy. 2010. "Water consumption increases weight loss during a hypocaloric diet intervention in middle-aged and older adults." *Obesity, 18*(2), 300-7.

2 - Boschmann, M. 2003. "Water-induced thermogenesis." *Journal of Clinical Endocrinology and Metabolism,* 12(88), 6015-6019.

Susan's Slim for Life Secret # 17 - Jump-Start Metabolism With EPOC

Excess post-exercise oxygen consumption (EPOC) sounds like a phrase for scientists. That's true, but what this "after burn" means for you is that if you do the right workouts, you can burn beaucoup calories even after your workout ends. Your resting metabolic rate will be higher all day, which will make it easier for you to lose weight!

After strenuous activity, your body continues to consume more oxygen (the way it does during activity) in an attempt to restore balance in the body's systems (digestion, cellular activity, muscle repair, etc.). The caloric burning is higher immediately post-exercise and gradually begins to taper off.[1]

High- intensity interval cardio workouts (HIIT) and long duration workouts have been shown to incite the highest EPOC levels. Sample water and land interval-training workouts you can use to incite this after-burn are listed in Appendix II.

Your interval workouts don't have to be super complicated. If you're a swimmer, after warming up, you can propel yourself through some sprint 50s with a rest interval in between. Or you can don an Aquajogger vest and run suspended intervals of fast running for 30-45 seconds with 15 seconds rest in between.

If you're training on land or in the water alone, music can be a helpful motivator. Music listening products you can use in the water are available at swimoutlet.com.

REFERENCES

1 - Borsheim, E., and R. Bahr. 2003. "Effect of Exercise, Intensity, Duration and Mode on Post-Exercise Oxygen Consumption." *Sports Medicine.* 33(14): 1037-60.

Susan's Slim for Life Secret #18 - Fidget Your Weight Off with NEAT

Maybe you know someone thin who never sits still. She's always in motion, waving her hands when she speaks, jumping up and down when she's excited, running off for another game of tennis or softball or golf.

They're the ones we want to hate—they seem to eat whatever they want and never gain a pound. But their secret to leanness is available to you and everyone else. Beyond the psychology of why we sometimes make poor diet and exercise choices, weight loss primarily boils down to getting the body to burn or utilize more calories than are consumed.

That thick slice of pie or handful of Doritos you see that annoying thin woman eating in the break room will be burned off in no time, because tennis burns calories, as does pacing and flailing your arms all over the place.

Mayo Clinic studies show that the number of calories a person burns during activities of daily living, also known as non-exercise activity thermogenesis (NEAT), affects a person's tendency to convert excess calories to fat. A study following 20 individuals showed that the obese individuals spent an average of 164 minutes more per day sitting than the lean participants.

Lean individuals also burned nearly 365 NEAT calories per day, which translates to a 36.5-pound weight loss in one year.[1,2] What this means to you is that a little fidgeting here and a little pacing the room there can make a tremendous difference in your weight over time.

This doesn't mean you should toss your gym shoes in the recesses of your closet. Regular exercise is crucial to your emotional, cardiovascular, muscular and bone health as well as an effective way to burn calories and keep metabolism high. But what you do in between your workouts is as important as what you do during them.

To take full advantage of NEAT, try the following: [1,2]

1 - If you don't need to sit, stand instead. You burn more calories standing than sitting. If it isn't necessary to lie down, sit up instead. You burn more calories sitting than reclined. Sitting for long periods of time is as harmful for your health as it is for your waistline.

2 – Walk while standing when possible (when talking on the phone, for example). Pace around, assemble or fix something, dust furniture or fold laundry when you talk.

3 – When shopping, instead of driving around for 10 minutes looking for a parking spot, park in a vacant spot further from the store.

4 – Take short walks after lunch or dinner. When waiting for a meeting or appointment, walk up and down the halls instead of dropping into a chair.

5 – Do your own cleaning and gardening as much as possible.

6 – Pursue active hobbies such as golf, bird watching, walking, kayaking, tennis, hiking, playing a musical instrument (standing), and swimming.

7 – If you must watch television, stretch or exercise on the stability ball during the program. Or instead of reclining, sit up.

8 – Use your hands when you speak—it will hold people's attention and burn more calories.

9 – If the fitness facility, luncheon or other event is within walking distance, leave your car at home and head out on foot instead.

REFERENCES

1 - Kravitz, L. 2006. "A NEAT 'new' strategy for weight control." *IDEA Fitness Journal*, 3(4), 24-25.

2 - Kravitz, L. 2009. "Calorie burning: It's time to think 'outside the box:'" *IDEA Fitness Journal*, 6(4), 32-38.

Susan's Slim for Life Secret #19 - Use Competition as the Motivational Carrot

Competition isn't for everyone, but for many people it can provide motivation to keep exercising or to step it up another notch. It's another form of goal setting. If you think you're too old to race, go back and re-read Slim for Life Secret #15 again.

Athletes more mature than 80 compete in running events, cycling races, swim meets and triathlons — accumulating medals and trophies that make their friends envious. Most active adult communities offer tennis and golf tournaments and some even have competitive softball and soccer.

If you have a competitive streak in you, use it to your advantage. When I joined U.S. Masters swimming and started racing, I dragged myself out of bed for 6 AM practice more often than I would have had I been swimming for fitness alone.

What if you've never competed before or you don't consider yourself athletic? Does that mean you should never turn out for a 5K run or walkathon? Definitely not. Once you participate in one of these events, you will see that people show up with many different objectives.

The myth of athletic competitions is that every participant is skinny, wears revealing clothing and runs a 6-

minute mile. Not true. As a matter of fact, at the events I have competed in, most of the competitors carried a few extra pounds and most finished in times that would be considered closer to a walking than a running pace. And they still had a great time!

Some people figure if they're not going to be fast, they shouldn't compete. Don't let your ego get in the way of enjoying yourself. I'm not the best runner, but I push myself harder with a group than if I'm running around the block alone. Even if I don't cross the finish line lightning fast, I can finish knowing I achieved a good workout that will leave me feeling energized and upbeat for the rest of the day.

These benefits more than compensate for any "embarrassment" I might experience due to my lack of running ability. I'm far more skilled at swimming, but that's okay. Since my husband and I participate in many athletic events together and swimming isn't his forte (unlike me, he's a really good runner), we each sign up for races in our weaker sports.

Many of my former clients in the active adult community of SaddleBrooke (in northwest Tucson) play competitive tennis or pickleball, compete in swimming races, or do triathlons. If you live in a similar community, most likely the HOA hosts a website that lists groups and training times.

The people I know at SaddleBrooke seem to be invigorated by the camaraderie, motivating atmosphere and excitement of competition (even those pre-race jitters and talking with others about them can be a little fun).

Competitive events come in all types. The most common include running events, walking or run/walk events, and cycling events. You can find U.S. Masters Swimming teams and competitions for pool and open water in your area at usms.org. U.S. Masters Swimming offers local and national competitions in most major U.S. cities. Groups such as Everyone Runs and Southern Arizona Roadrunners offer running races in the Tucson area.

Almost anyone who works out 30 minutes three or more days a week can finish a 5K run or a charity walk or even a short bicycling event. The trick is to find an event that suits your interests and abilities. If you can't swim lengths of the pool without stopping, the triathlon isn't for you.

However, if you have been in a rut with your training and know how to swim, cycle and run, mixing up your training with these three activities can be fun. Crossing training like this enables you to work more muscles over the course of your training week and reduces your potential for injury.

You can rest your upper body on non-swimming days and your knees and ankles on days you take to the water instead of running. Working a variety of muscles with these different training modalities can deliver an amazing looking physique.

If the word "triathlon" brings the word "Ironman" to mind, think again. Triathlons come in all shapes and sizes. The sprint triathlon is accessible to most reasonably fit individuals and, although distances vary, usually involves an 800-yard swim, a 12-mile bike ride and a 3- mile run. If you prefer swimming in a pool to a lake or ocean, there are races for you, too.

If you prefer mountain biking and trail running to hitting the pavement, you can give an X-Terra event a go. Many events for different endurance sports can be found at http://www.active.com.

Susan's Slim for Life Secret #20 - Derive Inspiration from a Role Model

Often when I'm working to accomplish a goal, I try to emulate the behavior of a successful person I admire. Some of my favorite role models are Al Jarreau (for his zest for life and amazing creativity; sadly he passed away on February 12, 2017), Michael Phelps and Dara Torres (for Olympic swimming and their amazing bodies) and Stephen King and Nicholas Sparks (for their discipline and writing achievements).

Stephen King's *On Writing* not only gave me a great deal of insight into King as a person, but outlined the writing habits that enable him to produce a tremendous amount of publishable work.

Watching Michael Phelps and Dara Torres swim in the 2008 Beijing Olympics fueled my desire to train harder. I was in awe when Phelps made a comeback and showed off his winning ways again in 2012 and 2016.

At age 54, Dara Torres has a leaner, fitter body than most women half her age. She was 41 when she competed in her last Olympics. Activity is as much a mantra for Dara (I've given myself creative license to refer to my heroes on a first name basis) as it is for me.

Even when Dara took a hiatus from competitive swimming, she never stopped being active and athletic. In addition to daily swim workouts, when she prepared for the 2008 Olympics, she poured her heart into strength training, core work, and stretching.

It thrilled me to hear she'd qualified for the 2008 Olympics and on a big screen after a day of racing at the U.S. Masters Swimming Long Course Nationals in Portland, I watched Dara win a silver medal in the 50-meter freestyle in Beijing.

Reading about her and watching her compete in the Olympics inspired me to reach my 2008 Long Course Masters swimming goals. As a matter of fact, I was so inspired that I obtained three personal best swimming times at the Masters championship, placing 2nd in the 100 and 200-meter breaststroke and 3rd in the 50-meter breaststroke.

Al Jarreau has been my favorite musician since I was 20. Listening to his familiar voice and his upbeat music has pulled me through some very difficult times. The optimism in his music always inspired me to live happy and to express joy and positive energy with others. I attended two of his concerts—exhilarating experiences both times.

There is something about his energy that you could just feel—that was so uplifting. The second one of Al's concerts I attended in Scottsdale was less than a month before he passed away.

Despite chronic back pain and other health difficulties, he only rarely stepped off the stage and kept stepping right back up there. He kept on touring the world, doing what he loved up until the very end. Music, performing, and uplifting others were his life.

The more I know about how other successful people work and live, the easier it is to construct my own strategy for achievement. During times of difficulty, I often think, "How would so-and-so handle this?" Emulating positive behaviors and lifestyles helps you get closer to obtaining the healthy and fitter body you've always wanted to have!

So how can my role models help you? I hope that you'll develop a burning desire to push yourself harder and achieve goals you might otherwise not achieve by emulating heroes and heroines you admire and can identify with. Look for people who are living a healthy lifestyle and that will inspire you reach your fitness, weight, and nutrition goals. If you read about their lives and how they achieved goals, you will find yourself wanting to emulate them.

I'll never win an Olympic gold, of that, I'm sure. But I can continue to swim my personal bests, just as Dara Torres has done. And why is that? Largely because I believe it is possible. Reading articles about her in *Swimming World* and *Sports Illustrated* and watching her swim on TV kept me excited and motivated.

I see some of her in myself. I'm a mom, too. I have a busy schedule. I do lots of cross training. I have been active all my life. And I'm swimming personal bests. We have a whole lot in common, and I feel her energy with me whenever I'm pushing myself.

Dara stays slim because the number of calories she burns in daily activities is equivalent to the calories she puts back into her body. The end result? At the end of the day, no excess calories are stored as pounds of fat on her midsection.

I've heard younger swimmers muse about how odd it is that Dara still trains hard at her age, as if after a certain age, one should slip into a comfortable sedentary state, parking oneself in front of the television with a beer and a bowl of potato chips. I admire Dara for her efforts and achievements — she has decided that staying in top physical condition is something she will do, not for a few years until she medals at the Olympics or wins the college conference championships, but for life.

I happen to be a very athletic person and so athletes provide a lot of fuel for my fire. Not all of you will find an athlete to be an appropriate role model. Choose someone who represents what you hope to achieve. It could be your neighbor who takes walks three miles religiously every morning before work or a movie star who manages to stay fit and trim despite a hectic filming schedule.

Susan's Slim for Life Secret #21 - Confront the Saboteurs

You've heard about people who deep-six the diets of loved ones. Maybe you find it hard to believe anyone would behave like that. Why would anyone actually want a spouse, daughter, sister or friend to fail at efforts to improve health? The answer is complicated.

Maybe your spouse isn't ready to change his or her eating habits. Maybe he's worried you will encourage him to eat smaller portions or reduce the amount of fat in his diet (he won't like it one bit if you identify his peanut-eating during the ballgame as "mindless"). A person feels more comfortable engaging in poor lifestyle choices when around "comforting" relatives and friends making the same mistakes. The dieter is about as much fun to a group of over-eaters as the teetotaler is to the bar crowd.

You may still be a little afraid of the changes you're making. But you have had time to think about it and to decide this is what you want. Some of your family and friends may be afraid of change and have not yet made a commitment to this change of lifestyle. They may worry what you're doing will make them feel guilty for sticking with the status quo or that you might become a different person if you lose weight.

Ideally, you can persuade the saboteur to overcome his or her insecurities and adopt healthier habits. In the real world, you will have to explain your expectations. Tell your spouse or friend there are wellness goals you want to accomplish and that you don't have any expectations for them to change, but that you do expect support for your efforts. If the person continues to encourage you to overeat or to miss exercise sessions, stand your ground! Don't cave in. Explain the importance of what you are doing and how this new lifestyle is important to your health and is now part of your identity. If the person really loves you, he or she will eventually come around.

Susan's Slim for Life Secret # 22 - Add Mung Beans to Your Diet

Most people unfamiliar with Ayurveda have never heard of mung beans, a legume in the same family as peas and lentils. Quite simply, they're packed with nutrients, reduce inflammation and improve the health of the digestive tract. I often throw them in soups. If time is of the essence, throwing a bunch of healthy ingredients in the crock-pot in the morning is a great way to return home after work to a meal already prepared!

You can also make kitchari, which is very healthy and easy to prepare. There are many different variations. Here is one way to prepare it.[1,2]

Ingredients

2 cups yellow mung dal beans

2 tbsp ghee or organic sesame oil

2 tsp black mustard seeds

2 tsp cumin seeds

1 tsp fennel seeds

1 tsp fenugreek seeds

2 tsp ground turmeric

2 tsp ground black pepper

1 tsp ground cumin

1 tsp ground coriander

1 tsp cinnamon

1 cup uncooked white basmati rice

2–5 cups of chopped, organic, seasonal vegetables (spinach, carrots, beets, sweet potato, squash, celery, kale, and bok choy)

 2 cloves

2 bay leaves

3 green cardamom pods

1 cup chopped fresh cilantro (optional)

Directions

Rinse and strain the mung dal beans until the water runs clear. In a large pot, heat the ghee or oil. Add the black mustard, cumin, fennel, and fenugreek seeds and toast until the mustard seeds pop. Add turmeric, black pepper, cumin, coriander, and cinnamon, and mix together.

Stir in the rice and beans. Add 8 cups of water, chopped vegetables, cloves, bay leaves, and cardamom pods. Bring to a boil and reduce to a simmer.

Cook at least one hour, until the beans and rice are soft and the kitchari has a porridge-like consistency. Serve warm with fresh cilantro on top, if desired.

Mung beans are rich in potassium, folate (Vitamin B9), Vitamin B1 and B6, magnesium, manganese, copper and zinc. They're also high in protein and dietary fiber, which give a feeling of satiety and reduce the temptation to overeat.

A study published in the *Journal of Nutrition* revealed that a single meal with high-fiber beans produced a two-fold greater increase in the satiety hormone called cholecystokinin when compared to meals that didn't contain beans.[1]

Because mung beans are so nutrient-rich, they are considered protective against diabetes, cancer, heart disease and obesity. They can lower LDL (bad) cholesterol, reduce inflammation, and scavenge free radicals in the body that can damage DNA.

Mung beans have a high carbohydrate content and work well for making flour and noodle products. In Chinese cuisine, mung beans are used to make pancakes or dumplings, combined with rice in stir-fries, and used to make tángshuǐ, in which the beans are cooked with sugar, coconut milk and a pinch of ginger. After cooking they can also be stirred into hummus or other dips or pureed to thicken soups.

REFERENCES

1 - Ingeborg, B., B. Olson, R. Backus, D. Richter, P. Davis, and B. Schneeman. (2001). "Beans, as a Source of Dietary Fiber, Increase Cholecystokinin and Apolipoprotein B48 Response to Test Meals in Men." *Journal of Nutrition.* 131: 1485-1490.

2- Levitt, A.J. 2005. *The Kripalu Cookbook: Gourmet Vegetarian Recipes.* Countryman Press.

3 – O'Donnell, K. (Author) and C. Brostrom (Photographer). 2015. *The Everyday Ayerveda Cookbook: A Seasonal Guide to Eating and Living Well.* Boulder, CO: Shambhala Publications, Inc.

Susan's Slim for Life Secret #23 – Don't Push Through the Wrong Kind of Pain

I've encouraged you to exercise often and even at a high intensity when it's appropriate. But sometimes when you exercise, you'll experience something worse than your heart rate elevating and simple muscle fatigue. Maybe you feel lightheaded or dizzy or confused. In these instances, you should immediately stop and if these symptoms don't quickly subside, you should call 9-1-1.

Sometimes you'll feel a strain in a muscle or joint during movement or feel pain in a joint such as the shoulder or hip. I've heard swimmers on our Masters team say, "My shoulder hurts." Between sets they grimace and rub the sore area, but they continue swimming for another hour. Anytime I experience something similar, I slow my pace or stop.

When you feel muscle pain that doesn't subside immediately when you stop exercise (such as a burn in the muscles you feel during a strength training set), you're experiencing strain or repetitive stress.

This is a cue from your body to stop. The best way to keep this minor injury from turning into a major one is to rest that part of the body for 2 or 3 days and apply an ice pack on it regularly to reduce inflammation. Regular massages can help alleviate irregularities in connective tissue that can potentially cause pain.

It won't serve you well to push through the pain. It will only put you at risk for injury, which could lead to you being unable to exercise or requiring surgery. This is not where the *Fitter Than Ever* program is supposed to take you!

One of the best ways to reduce injuries is to cross train. Engage in different activities throughout your week so you're not constantly over-using the same muscles and risking a repetitive stress injury.

Instead of swimming or running or cycling 5 days per week, swim on Tuesdays and Thursdays, run or walk on Mondays and Fridays, and cycle on Wednesdays and Saturdays (or assemble your own "different activities" combination)! Always include low or non-impact activities (walking, swimming, elliptical, cycling) each week. By embarking on cross training, you'll be able to exercise more with much less wear and tear on your body.

Susan's Slim for Life Secret #24 – Adopt a Dog

Research has shown that owning a dog enhances happiness, reduces anxiety, and improves overall mental health. Adopting a furry friend is also guaranteed to get you up off that couch! Your dog will depend on you for daily walks.

Taking your pet out will be a responsibility as well as an opportunity to exercise, enhancing your adherence. You'll bond during these outdoor treks together and both of you will be getting fresh air, moving muscles, and elevating heart rate for better health.

Susan's Slim for Life Secret #25 - Lose for Health and For You

This journey is all about you! Don't lose weight to look like a cover model or to please your family and friends. Instead of trying to fit into other peoples' concepts of what looks good (which usually leaves you feeling resentful and not wanting to do anything to change), set your own goals and embark on a journey to move toward them.

CHAPTER FIFTEEN
Pulling it All Together

You've nearly finished this book. I sincerely hope you've decided to make some changes and to start living a healthier lifestyle. I know the journey ahead can seem a bit daunting. Please, don't be afraid to forge onward. It's going to take work and commitment. But in the end, your whole life will change for the better.

Thanks to this book and your dedicated effort and commitment, you'll be able to spend more time enjoying life and less time at the doctor's office. Thanks to your efforts, you will soon have more energy, better concentration, and feel happier and more optimistic about your life. You'll also be able to do many activities you never believed possible.

You'll be able to attend your children's (or grandchildren's) athletic events and be able to walk out and back from the soccer field or the track without huffing and puffing. You'll be able to enjoy weekend hikes or bike rides with your family, not only for your own enjoyment but to set an example of a healthy lifestyle for your children or grandchildren.

You'll find your pants fitting looser and before long, you'll be ready to buy new clothes in a smaller size. Won't that shopping trip be fun to do with one of your walking or gym friends?

You'll feel proud of yourself when friends and people you meet ask you how you stay in such great shape. (When they do, of course, you'll tell them that a book you read by Susan Dawson-Cook really helped you change your life).

Most active adults consider their healthy lifestyle to be part of their identity. They might introduce themselves as a tennis or softball player or triathlete. I often tell others I'm a fitness and yoga instructor and competitive swimmer. Those activities that I do almost daily are a big part of who I am, as is being a mother, a wife and an author. Without my passion for the activities I enjoy most, I would be someone else entirely.

When you identify as an athlete, a swimmer, a golfer, an aerobics nut, or whatever, you will begin to feel as though part of you is missing when you are not doing the activity that has become an innate part of your daily routine.

When you get excited about trying new recipes and new foods, this quest to eat healthy will become part of your identity. It should give you a sense of pride and accomplishment knowing that your new healthy eating habits are reducing your risk for cancer, osteoporosis, diabetes, heart disease and other illnesses, which could slow you down and reduce your quality of life. And you'll feel a sense of freedom knowing you'll never again have to go on an uncomfortable starvation diet or be crushed when the latest five-minute miracle exercise plan doesn't work.

Because you're not going to diet and go back to bad eating. You're not going to exercise for a month or two and then collapse on the couch for a few months after that. This wellness program is going to become a comfortable habit— what you'll do today, tomorrow and for the rest of your life.

I believe you can be successful. Please have faith in yourself, keep employing these strategies, and the miracle you never thought could happen will come true!

APPENDIX I

Training Zones and Perceived Exertion Scale

Maximum Heart Rate (MHR) in beats per minute can be estimated by using the formula 220 – age (use the (210 - 1/2 your age) equation that I discussed earlier if you're over 50 and very fit). Depending on your medical conditions and fitness level, you can use that number to determine target heart rate ranges for one or more of the training zones appropriate for you.[1,2]

Zone 1, sometimes referred to as the "healthy heart" zone because it's often recommended for cardiac risk patients, is work between 50 and 60 percent of MHR. This low-intensity range is ideal for new exercisers and will enhance mood and burn fat.

Zone 2 is work between 60 and 70 percent of MHR and is a low to moderate training level. Work in this zone burns more fat and total calories than Zone 1. You should still be able to talk comfortably in this training zone. New exercisers (without health risks) should aspire to gradually work in Zones 2 and 3 as they get fitter.

Zone 3 is work between 70 and 80 percent of MHR and is a more challenging level that greatly improves cardiorespiratory fitness and endurance.

Zone 4 is work between 80 and 90 percent of MHR. You can work in this range for short bursts once you get fit if you're in excellent health. Training in this zone can help you to improve athletic performance.

Do not train in Zone 5 without permission from your physician.[1,2]

To obtain the low-end number for Zone 1, take your MHR number and multiply it times .5 to give you the value for 50 percent of your maximum heart rate. If you multiply MHR and .6, that will give you the upper limit for zone 1.

Here's example. A person aged 46 would have a MHR of 174. To compute the 50 percent of MHR number, multiply 174 by .5. This gives you a heart rate of 87. The 60 percent of maximum heart rate value is 104, meaning the Zone 1 range for this individual is between 87 and 104 beats per minute. You can follow similar formulas to get the ranges for zones 2, 3, 4 and 5.

Table 5. Zones for Training [1,2]

Zone	Percentage of MHR	Population
1	50-60%	New Exerciser/High Cardiac Risk
2	60-70%	Intermediate Exerciser
3	70-80%	Intermediate to Advanced
4	80-90%	Advanced or Short Intervals
5	90-100%	Athletes with Dr's Permission

If you are taking medication to control blood pressure, your trainer may recommend that you use perceived exertion to gauge exercise intensity. This is a method of estimating work effort.

Table 6. Rated Perceived Exertion (RPE) Scale

0	Nothing at all	5	Hard
0.5	Very, very easy	6	
1	Very easy	7	Very Hard
2	Easy	8	
3	Moderate	9	Very, Very Hard
4	Somewhat hard	10	Maximal

When you are at about a 4 on the RPE scale (somewhat hard), you should be able to talk in brief spurts without feeling winded. If you are unable to speak during exercise, you are working too hard. If you can give an entire dissertation of everything you've eaten in the past week or tell your friend everything that happened (or didn't happen) on your favorite soap or reality show, you aren't working hard enough.

REFERENCES

1 - Edwards, S. 2000. *The Heart Rate Monitor Guidebook to Heart Zone Training.* Sacramento, CA: Lifestyles Four Heart Press.

2 - Sachs, L. 2006. "Heart Rate Training." *IDEA Fitness Journal.* 8(6).

APPENDIX II

Interval Training Workouts

Do not attempt these workouts if you aren't aerobically conditioned or if you have cardiac risk factors. Always wear a heart rate monitor and never elevate heart rate beyond 90 percent MHR. Push yourself very hard during the "hard" intervals and track speed, resistance and RPM levels so you can note improvements. Avoid doing these workouts on back-to-back days.

35-minute workout - Treadmill/ Stationary Bicycle or Elliptical

5 minutes warm-up (easy)

4 minutes hard (speed) fast walk or jog

2-minute recovery (easy)

4 minutes hard (resistance) high incline

2-minute recovery (easy)

4 minutes hard (speed) fast walk or jog

2-minute recovery

4 minutes hard (resistance) very high incline

2-minute recovery

1-minute (fast speed) walk or jog

5-minute cool down

30-minute Track or Treadmill Interval running workout

5-minute warm-up (walk or easy jog)

Run at moderate tempo for 1 minute

Run at slow pace for 1 minute

Run at fast pace for **20 seconds**

Run at recovery pace for 40 seconds

Run at fast pace for **30 seconds**

Run at recovery pace for 30 seconds

Run at fast pace for **40 seconds**

Run at recovery pace for 20 seconds

Repeat the 20-30-40 sequence 5 more times

Run at moderate pace for 1 minute

Cool Down for 4 minutes

60-minute Interval Swimming Workout #1 (each length of the pool is assumed to be 25 yards or meters)

Warm-up 400 any stroke

4 x 75s (back, breast, free) moderate pace; 15 seconds rest

4 x 50s all-out kicking with board; 20 seconds rest

8 x 100s freestyle - descend 1 through 4 (each one progressively faster) and then 5-8; 15 seconds rest

2 x 200 Medleys - 1 easy, 1 hard; 20 seconds rest

8 x 25s all-out any stroke; 10 seconds rest

200 easy swim

TOTAL 2500 yards or meters

60-minute Swimming Workout #2 (can be done in 25-yard/meter or 50 meter pool)

200 swim

200 kick

200 pull

200 IM (50 fly, 50 back, 50 breast, 50 free) Drill

4 x 50s hard; 15 seconds rest, one of each stroke

6 x 200s Freestyle 1 & 4 - easy, 2 & 5 - negative split (second half faster than first), 3 & 6 - fast

200 easy

TOTAL 2400 yards or meters

75-90-minute Swimming Workout #3 (25 yard/meter pool)

Warm-up – 300 swim/300 kick/100 pull

8 x 50s – 25 kick, 25 drill

Main Set (do the set twice through)

3 x 100s freestyle on 1:30 (or interval with about 10 seconds rest)

3 x 100s best stroke on 1:45/2:00 (or interval with 10 seconds rest)

3 x 100s IM on 1:45 (or 10 seconds rest)

100 easy

8 x 75s kick (10 seconds rest), descend 1-4 and 5-8

100 easy

TOTAL 3800 yards or meters

APPENDIX III

Healthy Meal and Snack Options

Healthy Breakfast Options

- 1/2 cup Oatmeal with 1/2 cup berries, 4 ounces yogurt, 20 almonds (or see recipe for baked oatmeal below)
- 1 slice whole wheat toast, 1 tablespoon nut butter (peanut, almond, cashew), 1/2 cup orange juice, 1 hard boiled egg
- 1/2 cup whole-grain cereal (low-sugar) with 1/2 cup whole milk – watch out for granola which tends to be high in sugar.
- 1 cup of mixed fruit with 1/2 cup of whole milk
- 1/2 cup of plain whole yogurt with 1/2 cup berries and 10 nuts of choice
- 1 hard-boiled or poached egg with a slice of cheese and 8 grapes
- Whole grain waffle topped with sliced berries

Recipe for Baked Blueberry and Peach Oatmeal (modified from recipe found on http://www.emilybites.com); 9 servings

3 cups old-fashioned oats

1/4 cup packed brown sugar

2 tsp. baking powder

2 eggs

1 1/4 cup skim milk

1/4 cup unsweetened applesauce

1 tsp. vanilla extract

2 cups chopped organic peaches

1 cup fresh or frozen organic blueberries

1/3 cup chopped pecans

Preheat oven to 350 degrees. Combine oats, brown sugar, and baking powder in a large bowl. In a separate bowl, mix eggs, applesauce, milk and vanilla. Add egg mixture to dry ingredients and stir until blended together. Add blueberries and peaches. Coat baking pan with a thin layer of coconut oil to prevent sticking. Pour the oatmeal mixture into the dish, spreading evenly. Sprinkle pecans on top. Bake uncovered for 35 minutes.

Some Favorite Healthy Lunch Options

- 1 cup bowl of vegetable or lentil soup (200 calories - with chicken and broth)
- 4 mushrooms sauteed in 1 T. olive oil with a slice of cheese served with a half of an avocado (380 calories)
- Turkey sandwich (lettuce, tomato, mustard) on whole grain bread (300-425 calories, depending on condiments. Remember mustard and catsup have fewer calories than mayonnaise)
- Tuna wrap (380 calories) - make tuna salad with a 6 oz. can of tuna, 1/4 cup non-fat yogurt, seasonings (dill and garlic are two of my favorites), chopped peppers, and spinach. Roll into a wheat or corn tortilla.
- Greek salad (1 cup - 105 calories) with greens, tomato, black olives, feta cheese and olive oil/vinegar dressing
- Slice of thin crust veggie pizza (230 calories)
- Sushi (Tuna (184 calories) or Avocado Roll (140 calories)
- 2 slices whole grain sprouted bread, 2 ounces turkey slices, 1/8 of avocado, 1 thin slice of cheese, 1 cup of baby carrots, radishes, and bell peppers
- 1/2 cup hummus, 1 slice provolone cheese, 1/2 whole wheat pita, 1 cup vegetables, 1 small pear or apple

Many salads are easy to prepare and can be super nutritious. Some of my favorite salad ingredients include lettuce, kale, collard greens, feta cheese, tomatoes, mushrooms, beets, cucumbers, carrots, radishes, and avocados. If I want meat on the salad, I usually go for grilled chicken or salmon.

Healthy Dinner Options (Main Course)

- 3 oz. grilled Pacific Salmon, Flounder, Catfish, Sole, Trout, Tilapia, or Whitefish. Delicious served with whole-wheat couscous or Brussels sprouts.
- 3 oz. broiled or grilled salmon, 1 cup brown rice, 1 cup broccoli
- 3 oz. steak with 1 cup mixed greens salad with sliced tomatoes and cucumber
- 1 cup chicken fajitas with sauteed onions and bell peppers on a corn tortilla
- Baked or grilled chicken (remove skin and brush with olive oil and seasonings).
- Stir fry vegetables (possible vegetables - snap peas, water chestnuts, carrots, asparagus, broccoli, cauliflower, kale, mushrooms) with chicken or shrimp. Serve over wild or brown rice.
- 1 cup whole grain pasta with marinara and ground turkey sauce.

- 3 oz. grilled or broiled chicken breast, 1/2 sweet potato, 1 cup asparagus

Healthy Snack Suggestions

The right snack can take the edge off of your appetite (so you're less likely to overeat at your next meal), keep your blood sugar stable, and keep your metabolism up. When snacking, serve yourself the number of nuts, crackers, or pieces of fruit you intend to eat on a plate and then put away the package. This will prevent you from mindlessly nibbling from an open bag or box. These snacks are all 200 calories or less.

If you haven't read ingredient lists since you needed reading glasses, start now. You will be shocked at how much crap is in most snack foods sold in stores today. If you have health issues such as migraine or irritable bowel syndrome, you will feel much better once you steer clear of preservative-laced items. When you're feeling your best, you will be more likely to make better food choices.

- 2 slices of cheese or a a stick of mozzarella string cheese
- apple, orange, peach or nectarine
- banana

- 1/2 cup cottage cheese

- cup of diced papaya

- cluster of grapes

- 1/2 cup of blueberries, strawberries, or blackberries

- 1/2 cup plain yogurt with ½ cup fresh or frozen fruit

- 15 almonds, pistachios or macadamia nuts

 - 1 oz walnuts (~10 halves)

 - 2 tablespoons dried cherries, cranberries or raisins

- 1/4 cup of sunflower seeds

- 2 cups of popcorn (1 T butter)

- stalk of celery with peanut butter

- 5 carrot sticks with low-fat yogurt dip

Healthy eating shouldn't be boring or make you feel deprived. You can prepare delicious meals that are low in calories. There are many low-calorie cookbooks on the market today, such as the *American Heart Association Low-Calorie Cookbook: More Than 200 Delicious Recipes for Healthy Eating*, which offer ways to cook with less calories.

Even with regular recipes, you can cut calories by halving the amount of sugar called for in a recipe or making healthier substitutions (yogurt for sour cream, wheat for white flour [or coconut flour for regular flour if you have grain intolerance issues], olive oil for vegetable oil).

Printed in Great Britain
by Amazon